pure scents for
Relaxation

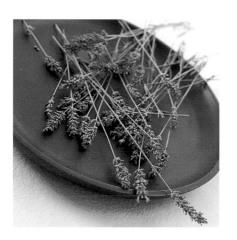

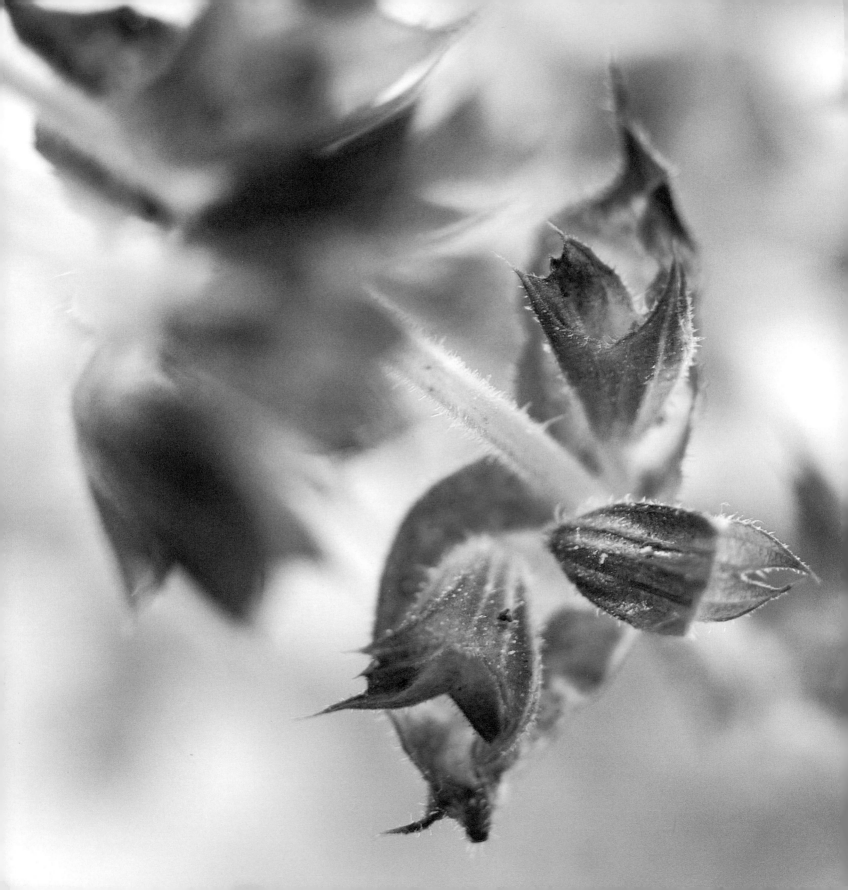

pure scents for Relaxation

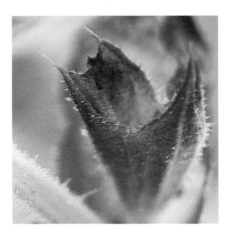

Joannah Metcalfe

photography by David Montgomery

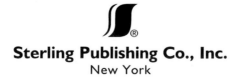

Sterling Publishing Co., Inc.
New York

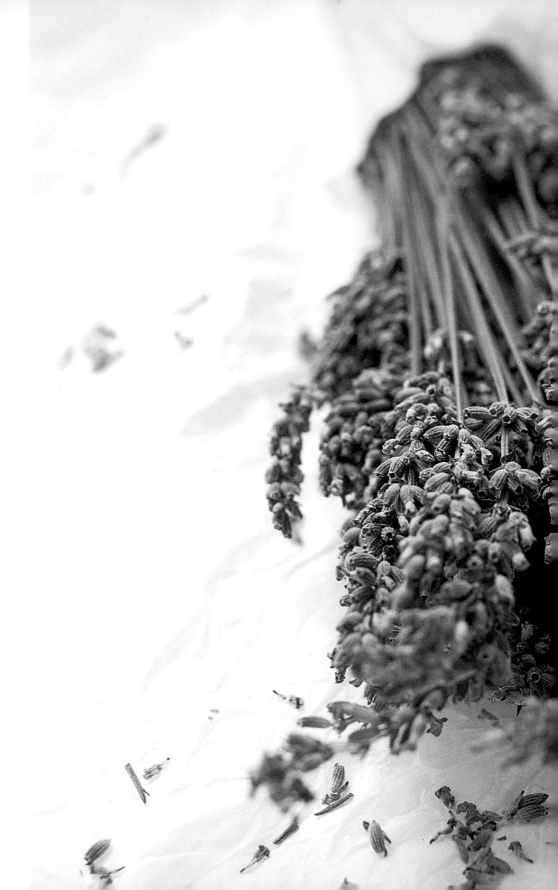

Publishing Director Anne Ryland
Designer Megan Smith
Editor Zia Mattocks
Stylist Sue Parker
Location Researcher Kate Brunt
Production Patricia Harrington
Author photograph Henry Wilson

For my daughter Harriett

Library of Congress
Cataloging-in-Publication Data Available

10 9 8 7 6 5 4 3 2 1

Published in 1999 by Sterling Publishing
Company, Inc., 387 Park Avenue South,
New York, N.Y. 10016

First published in Great Britain in 1999 by
Ryland Peters & Small, Cavendish House,
51–55 Mortimer Street, London W1N 7TD

Distributed in Canada by Sterling Publishing
c/o Canadian Manda Group, One Atlantic Avenue,
Suite 105, Toronto, Ontario, Canada M6K 3E7

Produced by Sun Fung Offset Binding Co., Ltd
Printed in China

Sterling ISBN 0-8069-4845-0

**Before using any essential oils, please read
Aromatherapy practicalities (pp. 74–5) and the
contra-indications in the Directory of essences
(pp. 76–8). The application and quality of essential
oils is beyond the control of the author and the
publisher, who cannot be held responsible for
any problems arising from their use.**

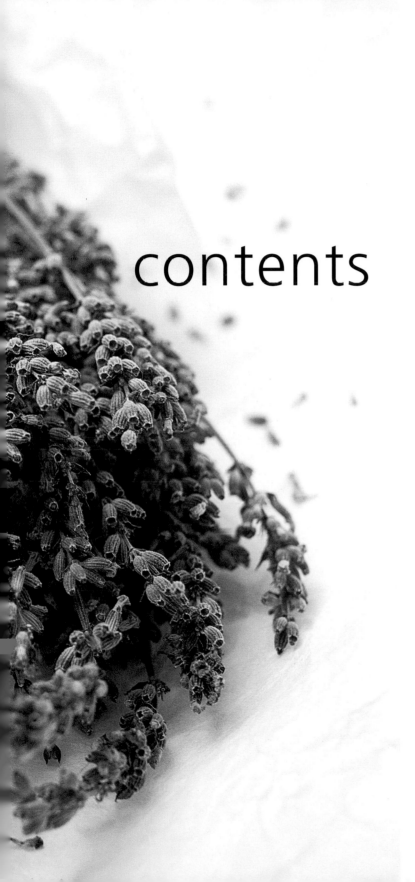

contents

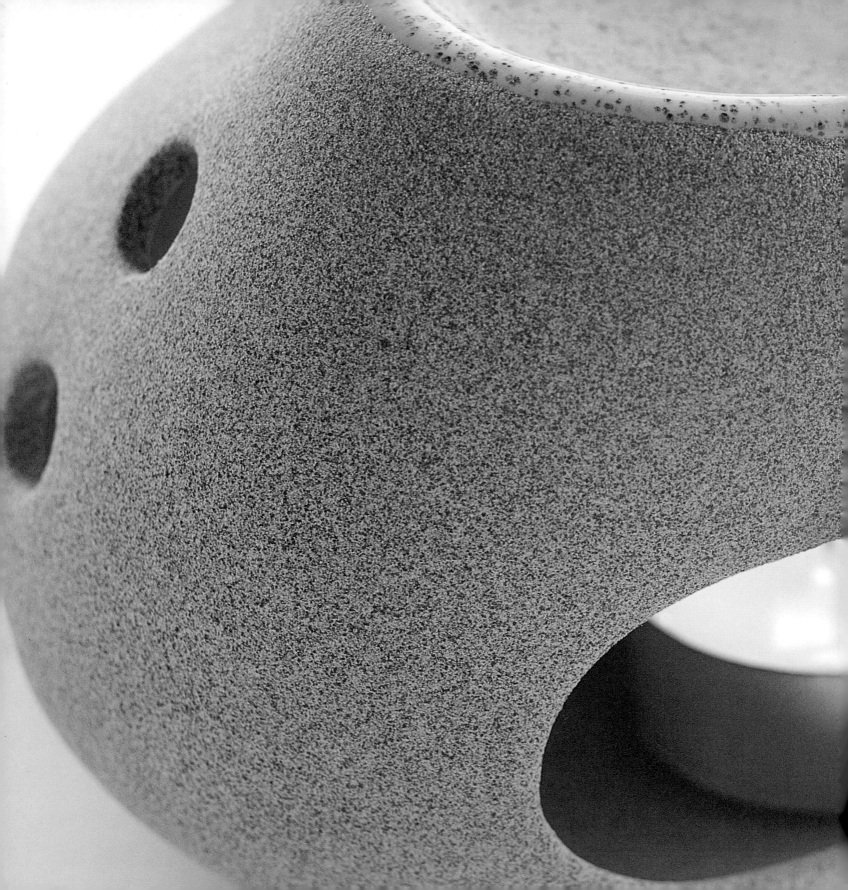

aromas for
RELAXATION

There are many natural essences with

relaxing properties that can be used

in diverse ways to soothe and pamper

a tired body, ease an anxious mind, and

create a tranquil, uplifting atmosphere

that will help to banish stress.

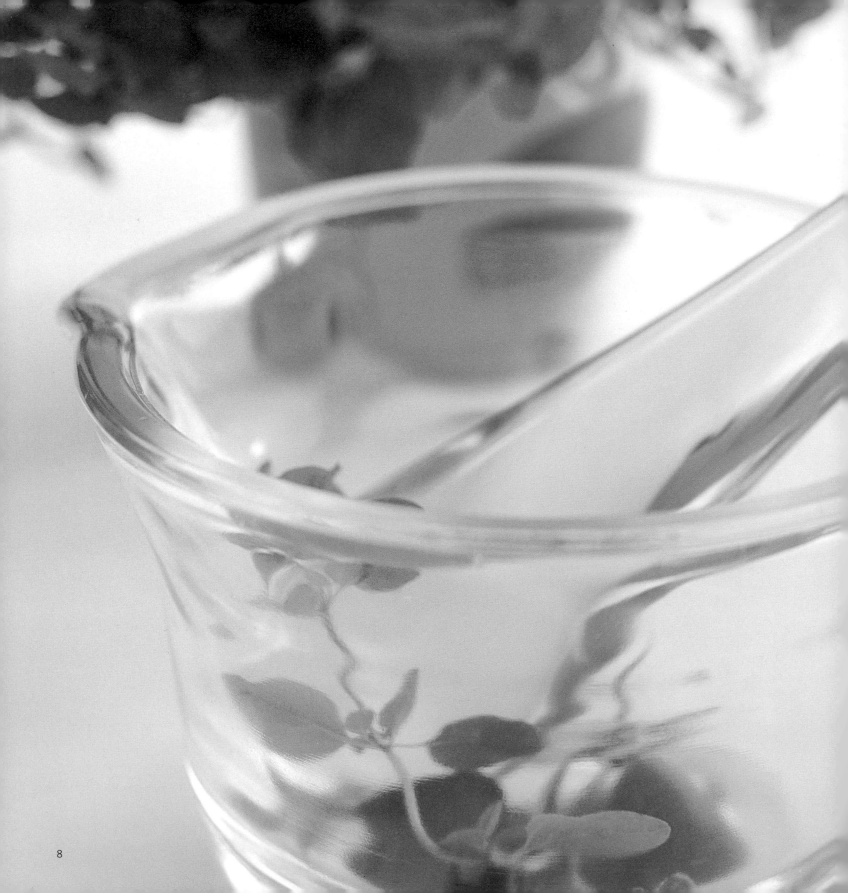

aromatherapy
past & present

Essential oils have been treasured for their beautiful fragrances, medicinal properties, and effects on the emotions for thousands of years. These properties, whether uplifting, sedating, or intoxicating, were probably first discovered by inhaling the smoke from burning aromatic herbs and resinous woods—the forerunner of incense burning. Reflecting on the use of essences through the ages gives us a greater understanding of the enormous wealth of knowledge we can draw upon and apply to great effect in modern-day aromatherapy practices, when, perhaps more than ever, we are in great need of what the essential oils have to offer to enhance the quality of our lives.

Far Eastern cultures have an uninterrupted tradition of using nature's provisions for many purposes. Both Taoists and Hindus used essential oils to enhance their spiritual, emotional, and physical lives. The ability of the oils to promote intense relaxation, deep breathing, and meditative states were used extensively to help access the higher realms within and achieve enlightenment. Their potential to help bring about spiritual transformation was held in reverential regard, and their medicinal and emotionally therapeutic effects were also recognized. The Chinese classified the essential oils into categories according to the mood they induced, all of which can be seen as aspects of the relaxed state: "tranquil," "reclusive," "luxurious," "beautiful," "refined," and "noble."

In Arabia, the philosopher and physician Avicenna was one of the first to perfect distillation techniques, which have changed little since A.D. 1000. Recognizing the link between mental and spiritual stress and low immunity and vitality, he strongly recommended aromatherapy massage to promote relaxation and improve health.

For thousands of years, different cultures around the world have recognized and utilized the multi-dimensional healing properties of many plants and herbs and the essential oils derived from them. The knowledge gained through the ages has gradually been refined and adapted for use in modern-day aromatherapy practices.

Ancient Egypt is considered to be the true birthplace of aromatherapy. The Egyptians greatly revered aromatic flowers and plants, and used them in all aspects of their lives. Beautiful water gardens were havens of tranquility, adorned with flowers from the distant lands of their vast empire. Especially prized were various forms of incense, which were made according to highly coveted recipes. These were used to alter and enhance moods, to scent homes, and to inspire devotion in temples. Creams, massage oils, medicaments, and perfumes were part of everyday life. One of the most famous forms of incense was "Kyphi," which contained a particularly relaxing, uplifting

Essences have been used for their relaxing properties for centuries.

combination of essences and was burned at sunset. It was said to aid restful sleep, relieve anxiety, and brighten dreams. Clothes, hair, and skin were perfumed with many exotic combinations, to lift the spirits and enhance the mood, for therapeutic purposes as well as to delight the senses. A special favorite for the relief of anxiety was "Therique," which was used as a perfume and in therapeutic applications for all manner of ills.

Knowledge flowed to other civilizations, notably the Greeks, who also recognized the mood-enhancing, calming, and uplifting effects that the essences imparted. They particularly favored flower essences, and used garlands of flowers around the head and body to uplift and revitalize those who were low, depressed, or fatigued. They used a number of relaxant herbs and oils, including opium, frankincense, myrrh, and rose. Hippocrates extolled the benefits of aromatic baths and massage to prolong life and vitality. He used herbs and essences for calming and relaxing the mind and body, and attempted to treat the causes of ailments, not simply the symptoms. The Romans also used aromatherapy in many aspects of their lives, particularly in massage and bathing. They greatly valued the relaxing, health-giving, cleansing combination of warm water and oils.

Exotic oils and resins, and the knowledge of their extraction were introduced into Europe during the 11th and 12th centuries by the Crusaders returning from Arabia. Essences were used mainly to make perfume to help mask the smell of the streets and to prevent the spread of infection. Aromatic plants like lavender and camomile were strewn on the ground so they would release their scent and therapeutic properties when they were stepped upon. Trade routes expanded, and the use of the more exotic oils and herbs swept Europe. Between the 14th and 17th centuries many books, "herbals," extolled the virtues of aromatic applications for physical and emotional problems, including the works of Nicholas Culpeper, which are still referred to today.

Paris had become the center of the perfume industry by the 19th century, and it was there that the link between scent and therapeutic effect was reestablished. The term aromatherapy was introduced in 1928 by the French chemist René Gattefosse, who discovered the therapeutic effects of lavender essence when he burned his hand working in a perfumery. He plunged it into the nearest liquid, a vat of lavender oil, and was amazed how fast his hand healed, without scarring. This stimulated great excitement, and aromatherapy began to evolve in its modern-day form.

calming, relaxing, soothing

The relaxing, sedative, uplifting,
or hypnotic effect gained from
inhaling the aromatic smoke of
certain burning plants has been
recognized and practiced for
centuries, for calming the nerves
and emotions, easing physical
tension, and aiding meditation.

origins of
essential oils

An essential oil is a highly concentrated, chemically complex substance, which is derived from the flowers, leaves, wood, fruits, seeds, or roots of plants and is totally natural in origin. The essential oils, which are highly volatile, are produced by one of three methods—expression, distillation, or solvent extraction. Expression, in which plant material such as fruit peel is simply squeezed, is the cheapest form of essential oil production. The majority of essences are produced by steam distillation, in which the plant material is placed in large containers and steamed at high pressure. The resultant water vapor, rich in essential oil molecules, is then cooled and collected. Very fragile flowers, such as rose, are distilled by solvent extraction—an expensive and time-consuming process—because in normal conditions the heat would evaporate the delicate molecules. The macerated petals or flowers are soaked in solvents and then centrifuged to separate the essential oil from the wax and other waste materials. This mixture is then distilled gently in a vacuum at a very low temperature to collect the pure fragile-flower essential oil molecules.

Camomile essence is a gentle, uplifting, hypnotic oil; marjoram has a strongly sedative action; while melissa, a very expensive essence, has a deeply calming and soothing effect on the emotions.

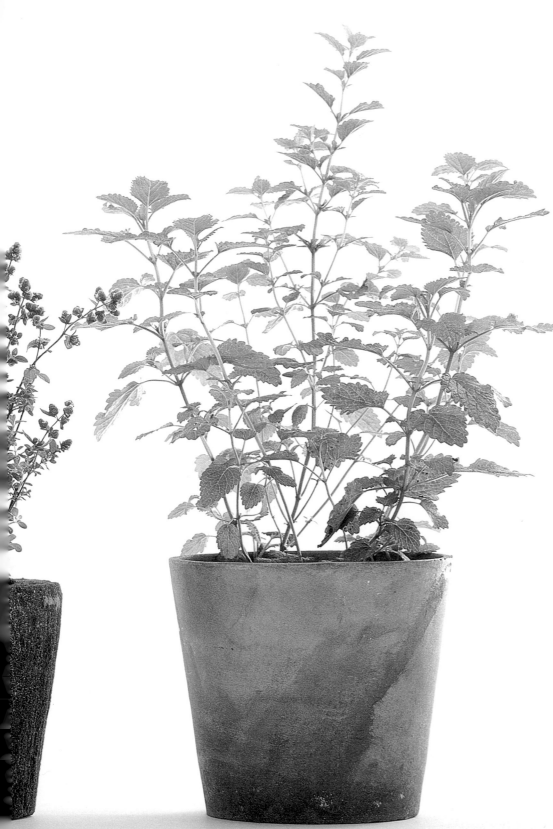

Essential oils can be used in many ways for their effects on the physical, emotional, and spiritual levels. They have powerful, nonaddictive, multidimensional properties, which can provide a valuable alternative to conventional drugs for many conditions, particularly for relieving the buildup of stress, tension, anxiety, and depression, which can affect all areas of life. Essential oils are particularly relevant to relaxation due to the calming, sedative, uplifting action that many of them impart. These natural effects in conjunction with the relaxing methods of application provide us with a profoundly effective means of counteracting stress.

The many ways scents affect us are as complex as the structure of essential oils themselves, and the study of olfaction has a long way to go before it is fully understood. This alone presents a strong argument for using natural products rather than their chemical counterparts, which could impart harmful side effects. Besides, while synthetic perfumes or air fresheners may smell pleasant, they do not have the antimicrobial, antiseptic, mood-enhancing properties of essential oils—and are often more expensive, too.

13

Essential oils enter the body by inhalation alone or by inhalation together with absorption through the skin. The majority of oils should not be applied neat, but should first be diluted in water, cream, or oil. As the vapors are inhaled, the molecules are taken into the capillaries in the walls of the lungs and conveyed around the body as the blood circulates, where they act according to their individual properties. Many oils also have antiseptic and antimicrobial properties that help relieve respiratory infections

inhaling & absorbing

Essential oil molecules enter the bloodstream either through capillaries in the skin or lungs.

and congestion. The part of the brain that deals with memory and emotions is connected directly to the lining of the nose by nerve receptors. As the essences are inhaled, this part of the brain is stimulated in positive mood-enhancing ways. Some oils stimulate and intoxicate the senses; others are calming and sedative.

For massage, essential oils are diluted in a blend of vegetable oils, such as sweet almond oil, olive oil, wheat germ oil, or jojoba oil. The carrier or base oil reduces the concentration of essences, prevents them from evaporating, and allows them to be spread over a wide surface area. It is a moisturizing, nourishing, lubricating medium, which enhances the external layers of the skin but is not absorbed any further, whereas the tiny molecules of essential oil pass into the capillaries in the skin and from there into the bloodstream and lymphatic system. The essential oils are absorbed most quickly through the thin layers of skin on the scalp and face, and the backs of the hands and feet.

Vegetable oils come from tiny glands in the flower petals, leaves, roots, or seeds. The majority—and the cheapest—are highly refined, which reduces their odor, color, vitamin and mineral content, and therapeutic effect. The richer, more nutritive oils can be added to blends, usually in dilutions of 5–25 percent, to help certain skin conditions, including dry or mature skin. These oils are rich in antioxidants, which help prolong the life of blends by slowing down the oxidation process; adding oils rich in vitamin E also has this effect. The best-quality vegetable oils are the cold-pressed varieties, such as wheat germ or avocado, but a high content of crude vegetable matter can be indicative of high levels of fungal spores, which proliferate if added to water-based creams. Therefore, these nutritive oils are best used in massage-oil blends and stored in dark, airtight containers away from direct heat. Don't be tempted to use synthetic man-made oils, as they will prevent the adequate absorption of essential oils, leaving your skin sticky, not silky, and they may also irritate sensitive skin.

Massage has a profoundly relaxing effect, and even without essential oils a good massage will release tension and spasm in muscles and encourage relaxation. An aromatherapy massage with essences specifically chosen for an individual's needs will multiply the effect many times over, and represents one of the most powerful methods of imparting a wholly relaxed state. Certain essences elevate the spirits; others help ease physical tension; some aid circulation and detoxification. The same blends can also be used in baths or inhalations, for vaporization, or to perfume bed linen and home furnishings to invoke a sense of relaxation whenever you need it. Used regularly, even as part of your beauty routine in natural creams or lotions, essential oils will help to relieve the buildup of pressure and stress.

Our sense of smell is highly sensitive, and a pleasant, relaxing aroma with a positive association will immediately help us relax. It is no coincidence that many of the supremely antidepressant oils come from flowers we naturally associate with summer gardens, such as lavender, rose, and geranium. Relaxing essences work in a number of ways, and their versatility mirrors their complex chemical structure and the many aspects of relaxation. The most commonly needed essences tend to be sedatives, such as marjoram, clary sage, lavender, and sandalwood, which help us to calm down and unwind. Hypnotic essences, which include camomile and neroli, are particularly effective for treating insomnia, while antidepressant essences are indicated when stress and anxiety have left us feeling low and lacking a sense of perspective—neroli, bergamot, ylang ylang, and geranium will help lift the spirits. Regulating essences, such as lavender, bergamot, and geranium, help to reestablish a sense of balance, both physically and emotionally.

The right side of the brain is associated with intuition and creativity, the left with logic and intellect. Usually, we operate with the left side dominant, but when both sides are in harmony, a sense of calm wellbeing is achieved. Studies of brain patterns have been made that prove the inhalation of essences has a balancing effect on the activity of the right and left hemispheres of the brain. It was found that when calming, antidepressant rose and neroli essences were inhaled, a brain pattern reflective of a meditative state was achieved, indicating the powerful ways in which the essences can help us relax and recuperate.

Although the uses of essential oils are many and their therapeutic properties affect the body on all levels, before you invest, bear in mind that oils from fragile flowers are expensive, due to the costly process involved in producing them. However, these oils are so concentrated they need only be used one drop at a time, so are sold in affordable amounts: 2 ml, 2.5 ml, or 5 ml. Most oils suggested for relaxation fall into the lowest price range. Melissa, neroli, and rose are the most expensive because it takes approximately 6 tons of melissa leaves and flowers, 1 ton of neroli

essentials on essences

blossom, and 5 tons of rose petals, which must be fresh and hand-picked, to produce 2 pounds of essence. Sandalwood, valerian, camomile, and frankincense are the next most expensive, then ylang ylang, clary sage, bergamot, and marjoram. Cheapest are lavender, petitgrain, geranium, vetiver, benzoin, orange, and mandarin: 1 ton of dried flowers yields 15–20 pounds of lavender oil; 275 pounds of leaves and twigs yield 1 pound of petitgrain oil.

Price reflects quality to a certain extent, and if you buy cheap oils, it is likely they will have been adulterated, either by chemicals, by cheaper essences (rose diluted by geranium, for example) or by vegetable oils. If you want 100 percent pure oils, check that the label or accompanying literature states that. Some favorite terms for impure essences are "aromatherapy" oils or "natural" oils. Essences sold in clear or lightly colored plastic

or glass bottles will not be pure, since they react detrimentally to light and corrode most plastics. Organic oils are preferable, since they will not be tainted by any chemicals; they can be a little more expensive, although some are actually cheaper.

Essences are affected by light, heat, and oxygen, and should be stored in a cool, dark place with their lids secure. Most oils keep for two years, depending how often the oil is used, since each time the lid is removed, it is exposed to oxygen. Oxidized oils look cloudy and should be used only for vaporization since the therapeutic action will be reduced. Citrus oils deteriorate at around six months (except neroli and bergamot, which can last up to one and two years respectively) due to the high content of a terpene element, limonene, which combines with oxygen. Some oils, like sandalwood and rose, improve with age like good wine. Essences diluted in a vegetable base that includes a small amount of an oil rich in antioxidants or vitamin E, such as wheat germ or avocado, should last for two to three months if stored correctly, but it is preferable to mix up small amounts at a time.

Use the essences individually until you are familiar with the effects of each, then try blending between two to five oils; more than five detract from the aroma and effect. Perfumes are divided into top, middle, and base notes, and the ideal blend includes one from each group—although this is a guide, not a rule. Of the 18 oils, top notes are lavender, petitgrain, mandarin, orange, and bergamot; middle notes are clary sage, geranium, lavender, neroli, petitgrain, rose, and ylang ylang; base notes are camomile, marjoram, sandalwood, melissa, valerian, frankincense, benzoin, and vetiver. Some are in more than one group due to the different layers of scent that give them a multidimensional character.

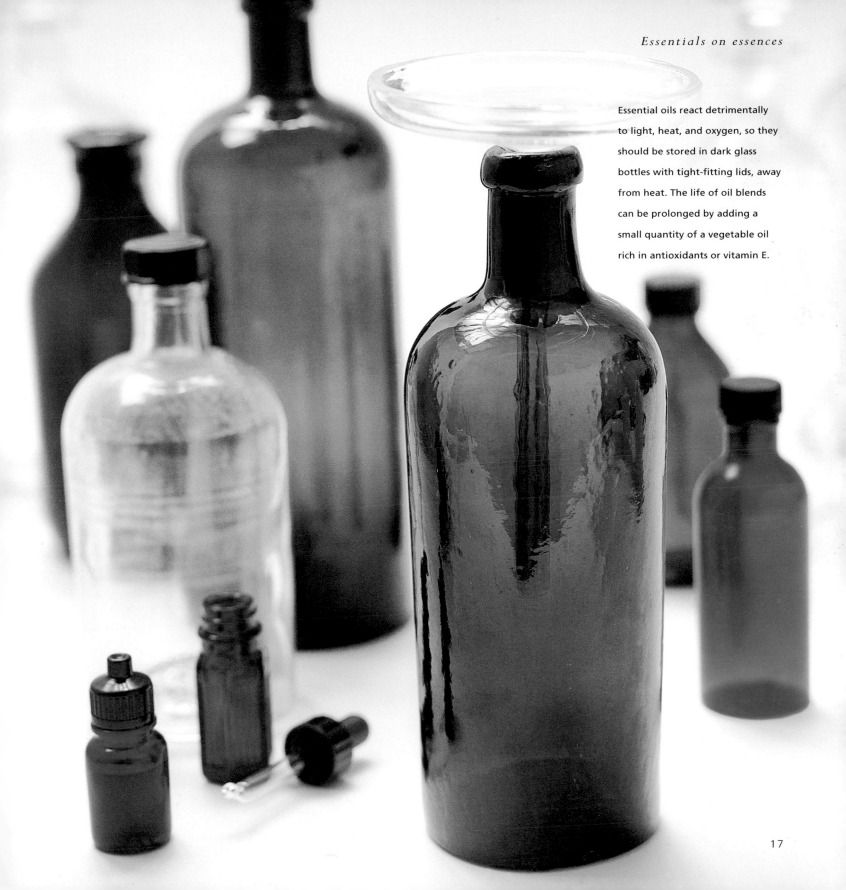

Essential oils react detrimentally to light, heat, and oxygen, so they should be stored in dark glass bottles with tight-fitting lids, away from heat. The life of oil blends can be prolonged by adding a small quantity of a vegetable oil rich in antioxidants or vitamin E.

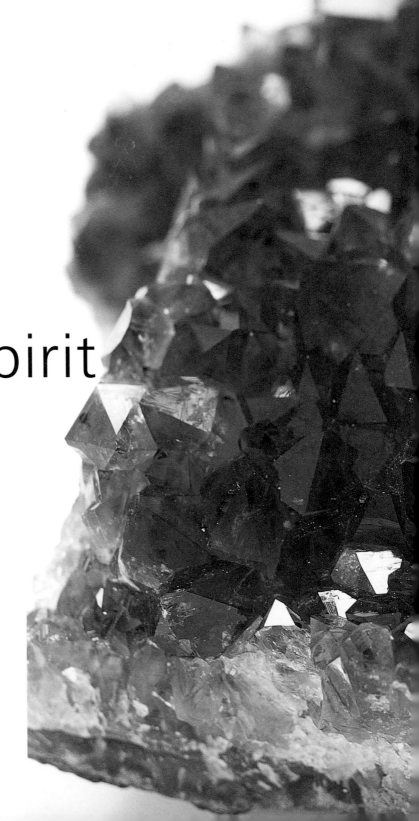

The fast pace and pressure of modern-day living allow us little time to call our own, and it is ironic that while our general standard of living is increasing all the time, many of us have less free time than ever to enjoy it. It is important to all aspects of our health and wellbeing to make time to establish a sense of peace and tranquility, whether we do this through tai chi, yoga, aromatherapy, contemplation, meditation, or crystal therapy, to help mitigate the effects of our stressful lives. All of these practices, on their own or in combination with each other, will help to relieve stress, tension, and anxiety, and promote our ability to relax and regenerate our minds, bodies, and spirits.

mind, body, & spirit

Whatever other relaxation technique you choose to practice, essential oils, which work subtly on the emotional and spiritual levels as well as on the physical plane, can be used to help create and enhance an atmosphere conducive to peace and relaxation, in which the thoughts can be elevated beyond immediate pressures or worries to restore harmony, balance, and a sense of perspective. Essential oils work on the emotions, helping to lift the spirits and encourage a positive and relaxed frame of mind, so we are able to enjoy our free time to the maximum and fully recharge our batteries. The deeply revitalizing properties of the oils themselves and the supremely soothing nature of the treatments make us more able to withstand life's pace and pressure and help us build up our inner strength.

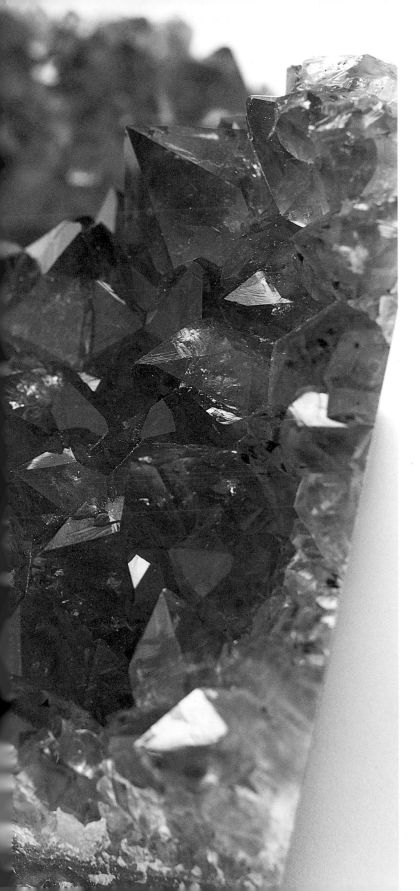

Crystals are mesmerizingly beautiful to look at and can help impart a peaceful atmosphere.

In addition to the many ways essential oils can be used at home, professional aromatherapy treatment represents a powerful antidote to many symptoms of stress and tension. Serious ill health can often be prevented, as long as we don't neglect our personal needs and wellbeing. Aromatherapy can help us establish a balance that lets us prioritize our lives more effectively and gain a clearer sense of perspective. It also means we devote time to promoting renewal and repair on all levels.

Crystals make ideal partners for essential oils. Not only are they extremely beautiful to look at, their complex molecular structure and the high rate at which these molecules vibrate means that they can be used therapeutically—and in industry—to transmit, enhance, and amplify energy. The energetic nature will vary according to the crystal's color, size, shape, and the way in which it is used and, as with essential oils, you will find you will naturally be drawn to those that will benefit you most. Crystal healing is a therapy of ancient origin, and crystals can be used to help enhance energy levels and create a relaxing atmosphere. Certain crystals have actions similar to essential oils and are related to them by their color or the nature of their action, and they can work beautifully in conjunction with each other: for example, lavender essence and amethyst, rose essence and rose quartz, camomile and blue lace agate.

Frankincense (below)
Boswellia thurifera
Warming, resinous, and mildly camphoric oil that is clear to very pale yellow, extracted from the bark. Blends with other resinous oils, such as sandalwood and vetiver, and citrus and floral oils. *Sedative, warming, regenerating.*

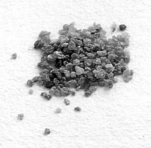

Sandalwood (not shown)
Santalum album
Warm, woody oil, which varies from pale yellow to dark brown, extracted from the roots and heartwood. Blends with benzoin, vetiver, clary sage, citrus, and floral oils, especially bergamot, neroli, rose, geranium, and lavender. *Antidepressant, aphrodisiac, sedative, antiseptic, emollient.*

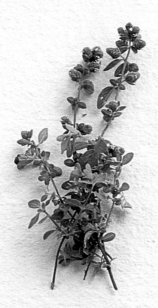

Marjoram (left)
Origanum majorana
Pale yellow oil that has a warm, sweet, herbaceous scent with a hint of camphor and pepper, extracted from the flowers and leaves. Blends especially well with camomile and lavender. *Strongly sedative, analgesic, antispasmodic.*

Bergamot (not shown)
Citrus bergamia
The light green oil is fresh, sweet, and citrus with floral undertones, extracted from the rind of the fruit. Blends with sandalwood, benzoin, camomile, frankincense, and clary sage, and floral oils, especially geranium, lavender, neroli, and ylang ylang. *Antidepressant, antimicrobial, refreshing, harmonizing.*

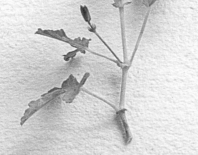

Geranium (left)
Pelargonium graveolens
Strong, sweet, slightly floral, pale green oil, extracted from the flowers and leaves. Blends with virtually all oils, especially lavender, rose, neroli, bergamot, clary sage, petitgrain, sandal-wood, and frankincense. *Balancing, refreshing, antidepressant, diuretic.*

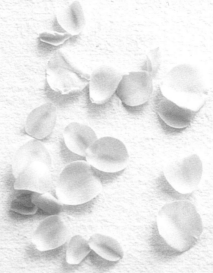

Rose (left)
Rosa damascena
Gorgeous, feminine, intensely sweet floral oil that is colorless to pale yellow, extracted from the petals. Blends with all oils, especially citrus essences, sandalwood, and geranium. *Antidepressant, aphrodisiac, nerve, heart, and digestive tonic.*

relaxing essences

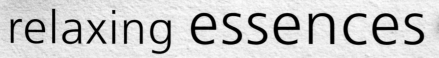

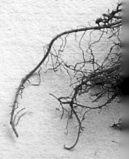

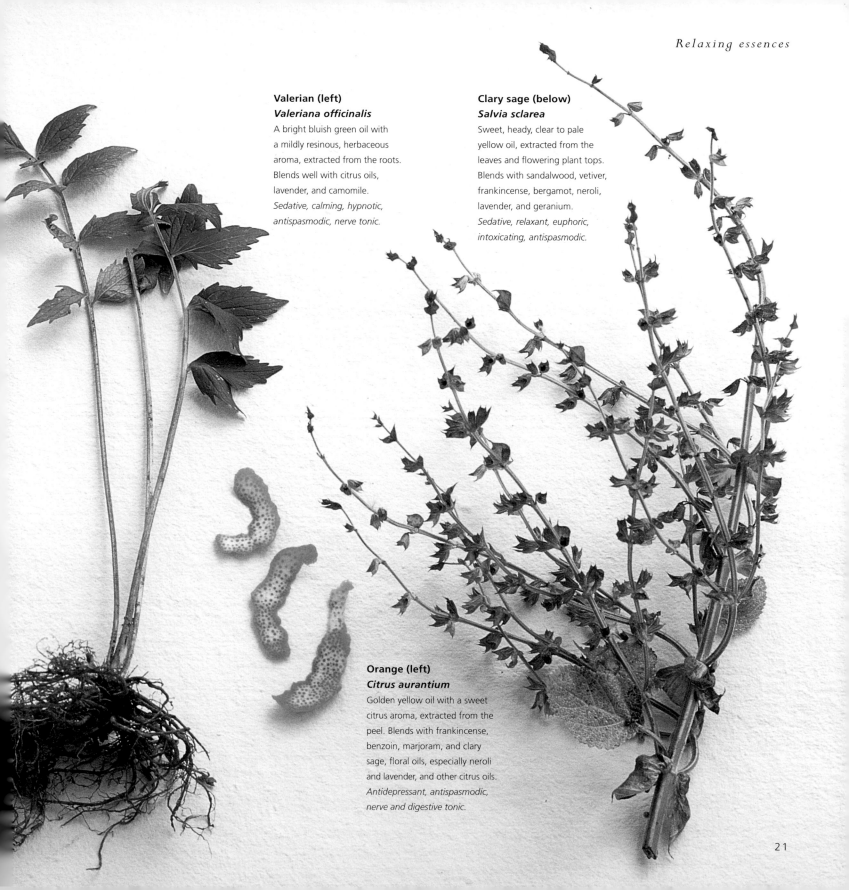

Valerian (left)
Valeriana officinalis
A bright bluish green oil with
a mildly resinous, herbaceous
aroma, extracted from the roots.
Blends well with citrus oils,
lavender, and camomile.
Sedative, calming, hypnotic,
antispasmodic, nerve tonic.

Clary sage (below)
Salvia sclarea
Sweet, heady, clear to pale
yellow oil, extracted from the
leaves and flowering plant tops.
Blends with sandalwood, vetiver,
frankincense, bergamot, neroli,
lavender, and geranium.
Sedative, relaxant, euphoric,
intoxicating, antispasmodic.

Orange (left)
Citrus aurantium
Golden yellow oil with a sweet
citrus aroma, extracted from the
peel. Blends with frankincense,
benzoin, marjoram, and clary
sage, floral oils, especially neroli
and lavender, and other citrus oils.
Antidepressant, antispasmodic,
nerve and digestive tonic.

21

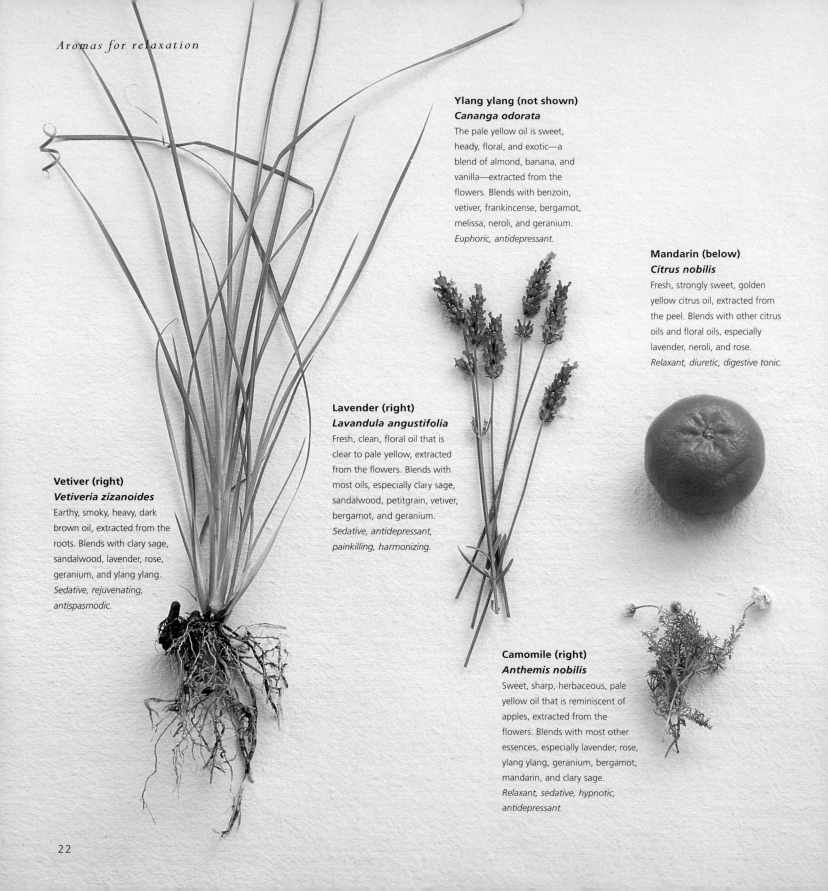

Ylang ylang (not shown)
Cananga odorata
The pale yellow oil is sweet, heady, floral, and exotic—a blend of almond, banana, and vanilla—extracted from the flowers. Blends with benzoin, vetiver, frankincense, bergamot, melissa, neroli, and geranium. *Euphoric, antidepressant.*

Mandarin (below)
Citrus nobilis
Fresh, strongly sweet, golden yellow citrus oil, extracted from the peel. Blends with other citrus oils and floral oils, especially lavender, neroli, and rose. *Relaxant, diuretic, digestive tonic.*

Lavender (right)
Lavandula angustifolia
Fresh, clean, floral oil that is clear to pale yellow, extracted from the flowers. Blends with most oils, especially clary sage, sandalwood, petitgrain, vetiver, bergamot, and geranium. *Sedative, antidepressant, painkilling, harmonizing.*

Vetiver (right)
Vetiveria zizanoides
Earthy, smoky, heavy, dark brown oil, extracted from the roots. Blends with clary sage, sandalwood, lavender, rose, geranium, and ylang ylang. *Sedative, rejuvenating, antispasmodic.*

Camomile (right)
Anthemis nobilis
Sweet, sharp, herbaceous, pale yellow oil that is reminiscent of apples, extracted from the flowers. Blends with most other essences, especially lavender, rose, ylang ylang, geranium, bergamot, mandarin, and clary sage. *Relaxant, sedative, hypnotic, antidepressant.*

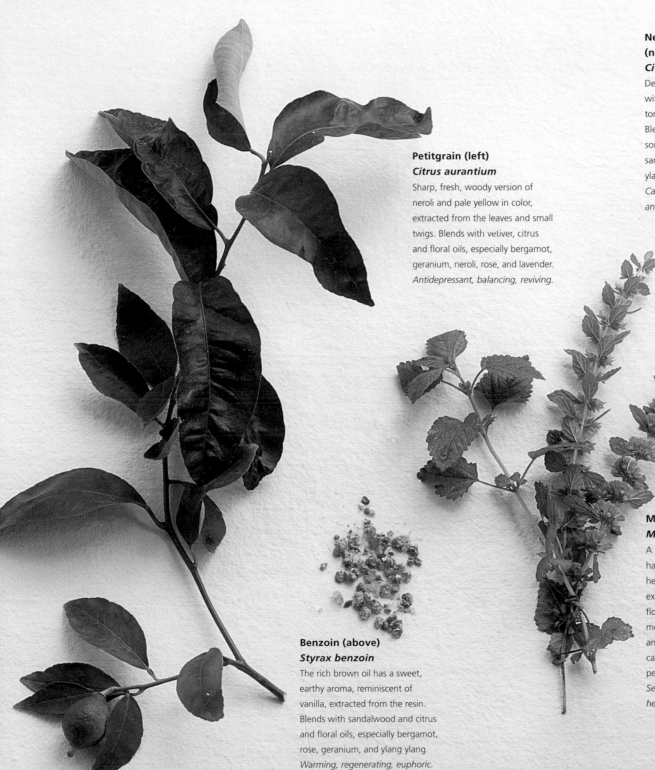

Neroli, orange blossom (not shown)
Citrus aurantium
Delicious pale yellow floral oil with bitter, slightly spicy under-tones, extracted from the flowers. Blends with floral, citrus, and some resinous oils, especially sandalwood, bergamot, ylang ylang, clary sage, and geranium. *Calming, sedative, hypnotic, antidepressant, regenerating.*

Petitgrain (left)
Citrus aurantium
Sharp, fresh, woody version of neroli and pale yellow in color, extracted from the leaves and small twigs. Blends with veliver, citrus and floral oils, especially bergamot, geranium, neroli, rose, and lavender. *Antidepressant, balancing, reviving.*

Melissa (left)
Melissa officinalis
A dark greenish yellow oil that has a heavy lemony scent with herbaceous honeylike overtones, extracted from the leaves and flowering plant tops. Blends with most essences, especially floral and citrus oils, such as lavender, camomile, geranium, neroli, petitgrain, and bergamot. *Sedative, antidepressant, nerve, heart, and digestive tonic.*

Benzoin (above)
Styrax benzoin
The rich brown oil has a sweet, earthy aroma, reminiscent of vanilla, extracted from the resin. Blends with sandalwood and citrus and floral oils, especially bergamot, rose, geranium, and ylang ylang. *Warming, regenerating, euphoric.*

23

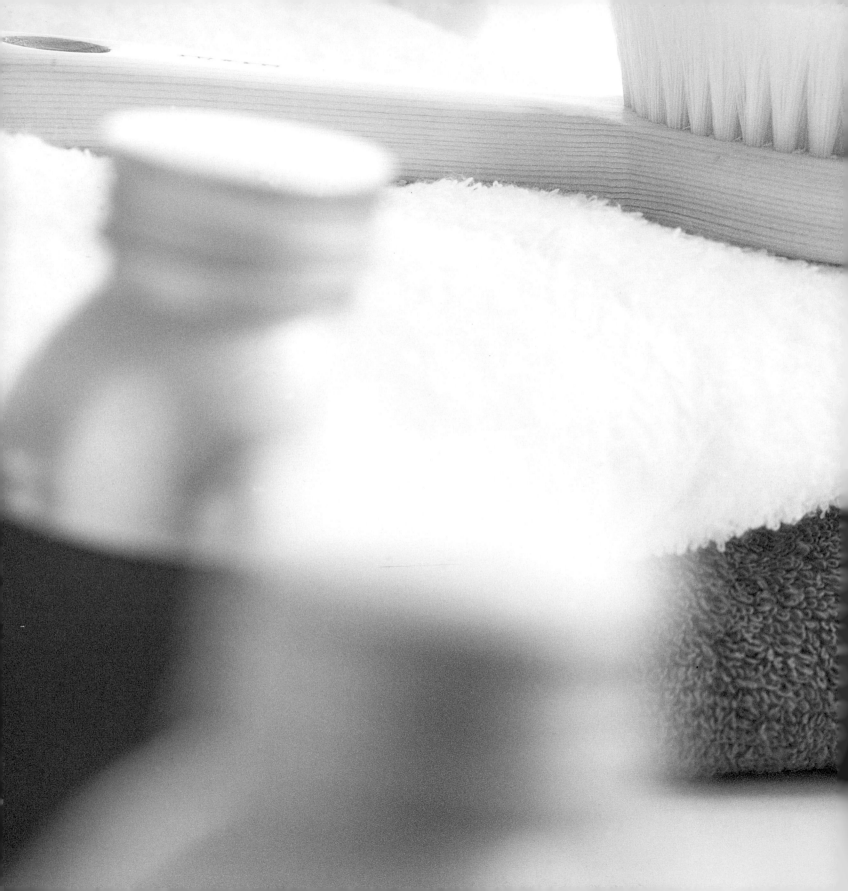

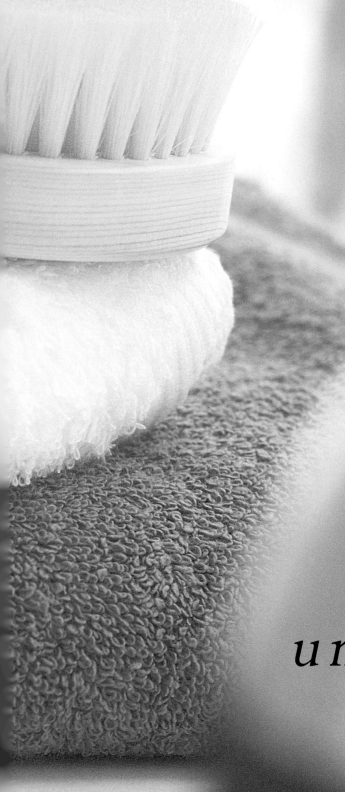

Counteract the stressful effects of a high-pressure job or hectic lifestyle, using the most soothing essences in baths, massage, and beauty treatments to help relax the body and mind.

unwind the
BODY

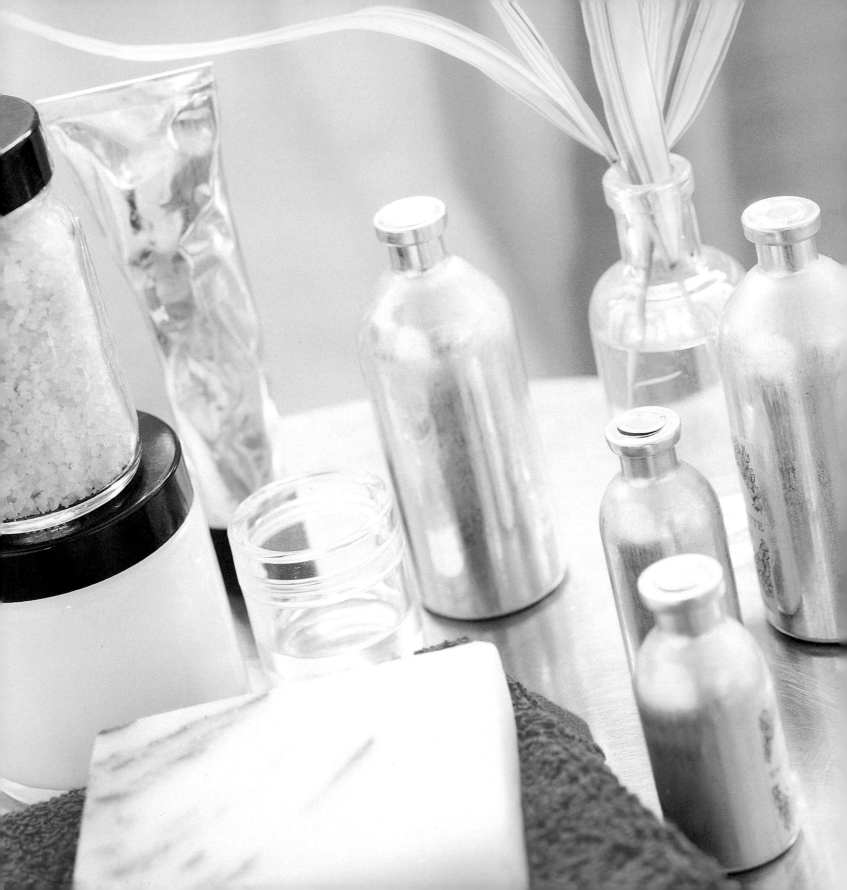

Taking a holistic approach to relaxation is paramount, since there are many areas of our lives other than those relating to the pressures of work or obvious responsibilities that can have a strong influence on our ability to unwind, such as our diet, exercise regime (or lack of it), and sleep pattern. Whatever form tension and stress take, essential oils can be used to help

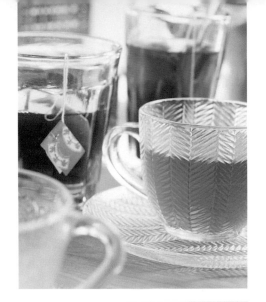

pampering the body on

the inside & outside

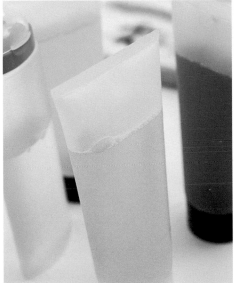

redress the balance. Their natural, gentle, yet powerful action in combination with their versatility of application—in soothing beauty treatments, relaxing massages, and calming aromatic baths—makes them a perfect choice for pampering a tired body and restoring a sense of peace, perspective, and balance.

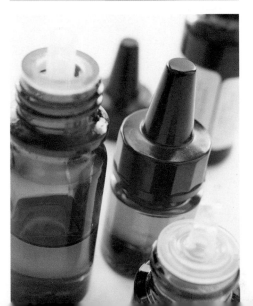

Tension affects us mentally and physically and manifests itself in different ways, perhaps the most damaging in the long term being an inability to relax and rest. Whatever pressures we experience, a difficulty in switching off mentally can be a precursor to many health problems and erode our quality of life. Stress-related symptoms include anything from head-aches and high blood pressure to heart attacks, so looking at ways to increase our ability to relax and revitalize ourselves is sure to be beneficial on every level.

An inability to relax can be detri-mental to our body in many ways. It affects the cells' ability to repair and renew themselves; our ability to digest food efficiently and absorb nutrients successfully; the standard and strength of our immune system's response to infection; and our general state of health. It also limits our capacity to retain information and maintain concentration when working under pressure, and reduces the strength of our libido.

Analyzing the level of stress from which you suffer can be a helpful first step in training yourself to relax and in choosing the essential oils and the

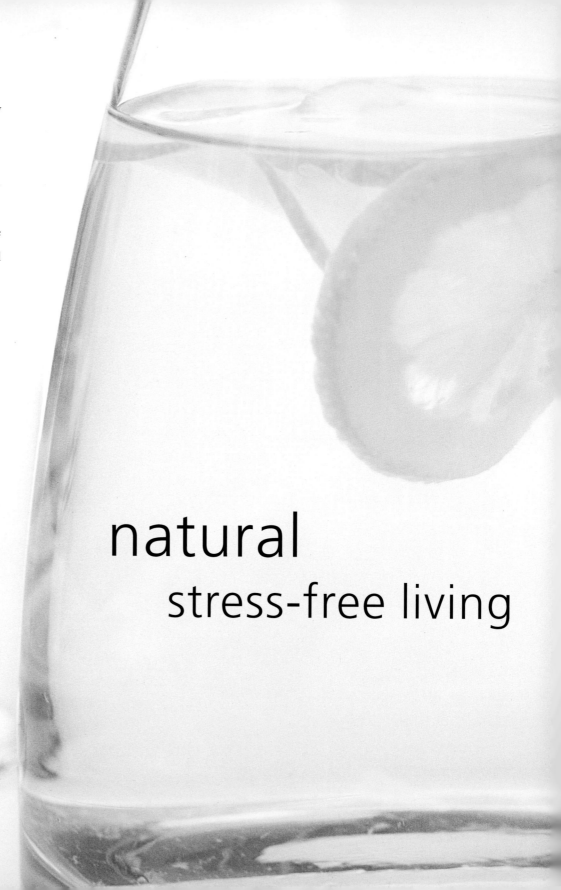

natural
stress-free living

applications that are most appropriate for your needs. One of the most significant indications of which oils you should use are the ones you like best, since the body naturally draws you to what it recognizes will be of most benefit.

Moderate stress can be caused by any aspect of a full life: driving in busy traffic; responsibilities at home or work; arguments with loved ones; not having enough time to achieve your day-to-day goals. This can result in the sort of complaints most people suffer from occasionally: headaches; mild infections; aches in the neck, shoulder, or back; and bouts of anxiety or frustration.

Chronic stress—a more long-term condition—may result if you have a high-pressure job, relationship difficulties, money problems, lack of sleep, poor time management, or lack of control over a situation at work or home. This can lead to regular back or neck pain, headaches, migraines, infections, digestive problems, high blood pressure, irregular periods, constant tiredness, and mood swings. These are our body's early warnings and should not be ignored, but should prompt us to seek professional help before we have a serious problem on our hands. It is important to recognize that even if we believe we are able to withstand these symptoms in the short term, we may suffer repercussions later.

Acute stress may result from a sudden shock, such as a relationship breakdown, bereavement, house move, job loss, accident, hospitalization, or a general feeling of being out of control. Symptoms may be severe migraine, neck or back pain, chronic exhaustion, severe skin conditions, panic attacks, irritable bowel syndrome, a duodenal or stomach ulcer; in the worst cases it may even lead to a breakdown, heart attack, or stroke. Using essential oils will help to ease some of these symptoms, but obviously professional help should be sought.

Bach Flower Remedies' "Rescue Remedy" is often recommended by complementary practitioners to help relieve stress and can be used alongside aromatherapy. Perhaps the most important thing for all aspects of health is to drink at least 2 pints of pure water a day to help detoxify, regenerate, and rejuvenate the system; it also helps clear the skin and prevent headaches and dehydration.

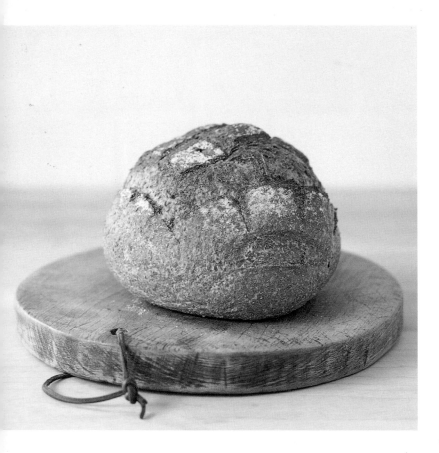

nourishing
the body

Many people do not realize the vital role diet plays in our ability to cope with stress and our capacity to relax and recuperate. When we are under pressure, fight-or-flight hormones are released into the bloodstream to enable us to rise to the occasion. These are of great use for the time we require them, but are often still present when we no longer need them, especially if we consume food that stimulates their release, preventing us from relaxing and ultimately having a detrimental effect on our health. Tea, coffee, alcohol, cola, chocolate, and refined carbohydrates contain high levels of caffeine and other chemicals that can cause health problems, offering our bodies little nutritional value in return for all the stress and strain they experience.

A stressful lifestyle causes vitamins and minerals to be used up more quickly than normal, often the ones we have most need of in stressful situations, such as vitamin B complex, vitamin C, calcium, magnesium, and zinc. It may be advisable to supplement your intake of these nutrients when you are under stress to help prevent "burnout" symptoms or, if you prefer, eat more fresh fruit and vegetables (raw, lightly steamed, or stir-fried, not boiled); whole-grain cereals and bread; dried peas and beans (cooked); rice and pasta; low-fat milk, yogurt or soybean products; lean white meat and fish (especially oily fish like herring, salmon, mackerel, and sardines). Eat organic or free-range food where possible to reduce the intake of toxins and avoid high levels of sugar, highly refined food, and artificial sweeteners, flavorings, preservatives, and colorants. Chew food well to aid digestion, and don't go for long periods without eating, as this strains the system. Even a very healthy meal just before bed can prevent relaxation and peaceful sleep.

A good source of fiber is whole-grain bread, which contains more goodness than refined white bread. Fresh fruit juices, rich in vitamin C, are healthy alternatives to many sugary or caffeine-laden drinks, which have little nutritional value.

Limit your daily intake of coffee and tea to three cups and don't regularly drink more than three units of alcohol, since it is a strong stimulant that is thought to increase predisposition to nutritional deficiencies and some forms of cancer.

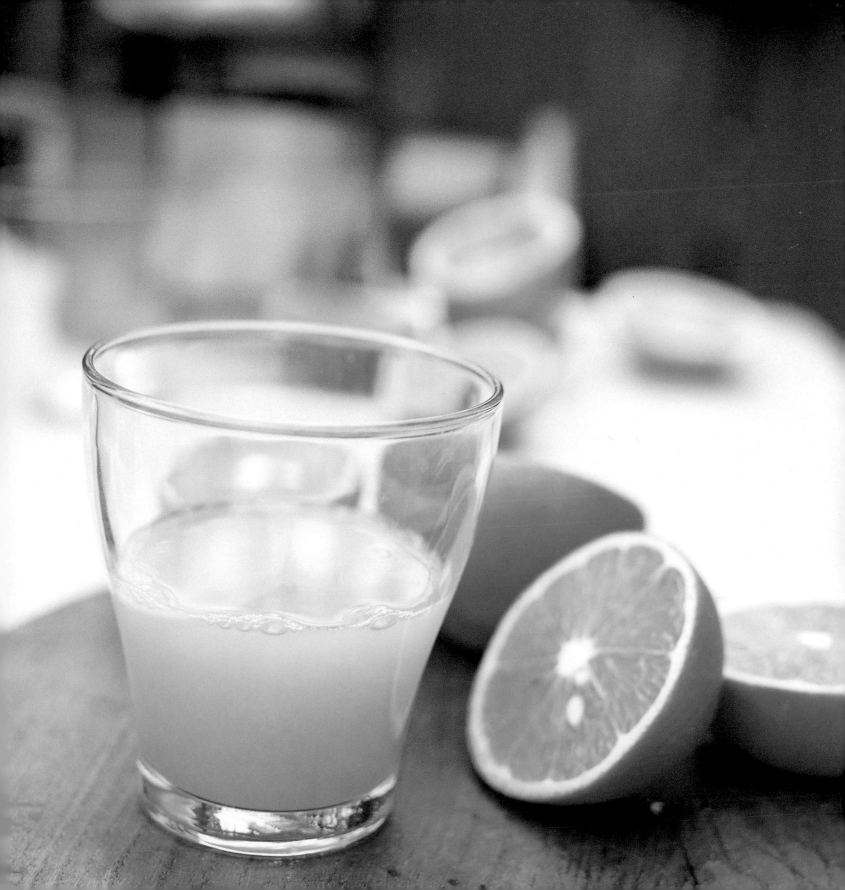

Herbal teas are far better for you than regular tea or coffee, which both contain high levels of caffeine. A bedtime drink of camomile tea, in particular, helps encourage peaceful sleep, and hops also make a naturally sedative tea. Each infusion should be allowed to steep for at least five minutes; add honey to your own taste. A glass of warm milk, with a little honey and nutmeg, will also help promote rest, since calcium soothes the nerves and heat speeds up the digestive process.

herbal tea
infusions

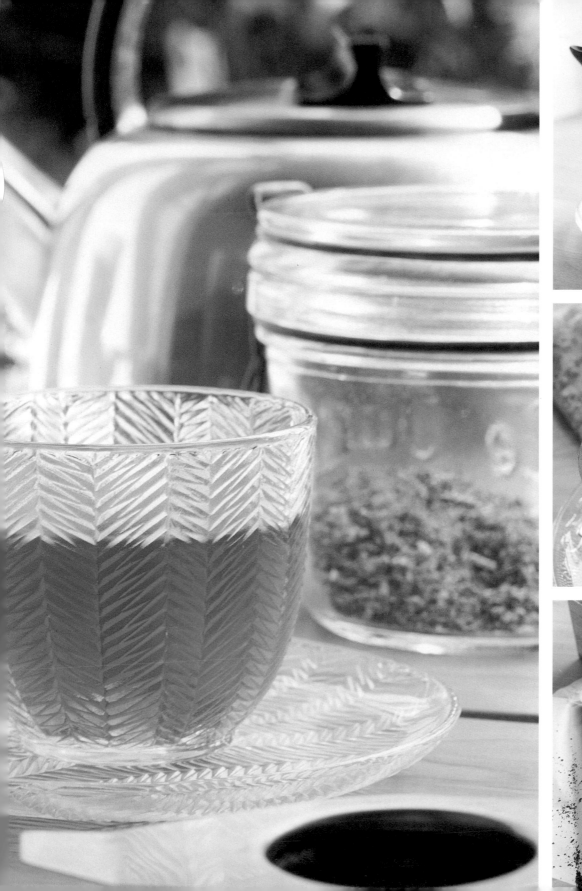
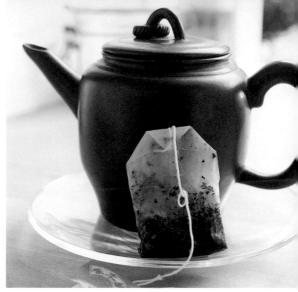
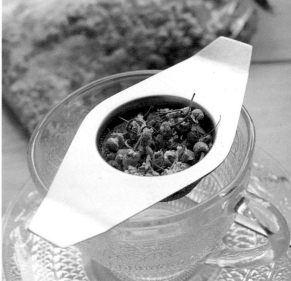
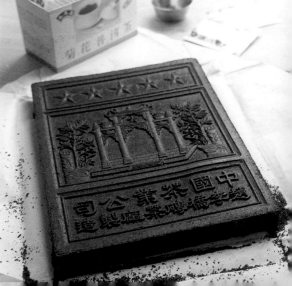

oil blends

Pre-exercise massage oil

To loosen muscles and help prevent strain, add to 2 tablespoons base oil:

Lavender essence, 5 drops

Frankincense essence, 3 drops

Benzoin essence, 1 drop

Post-exercise massage oil

To relax muscles and prevent stiffness, add to 2 tablespoons base oil:

Lavender essence, 8 drops

Clary sage essence, 4 drops

Camomile essence, 1 drop

For muscular aches and pains

To relieve strained muscles, add to 2 tablespoons base oil:

Marjoram essence, 6 drops

Camomile essence, 2 drops

Vetiver essence, 1 drop

Compress for a strain or spasm

Fill 1 bowl with hot water and 1 with cold water, then add to each:

Lavender essence, 6 drops

Vetiver essence, 1 drop

Camomile essence, 1 drop

Soak a square of fabric in each bowl; squeeze and apply alternately at 2-minute intervals. Repeat for 30 minutes or until discomfort is eased.

For properties of base oils *see* p. 40.

34

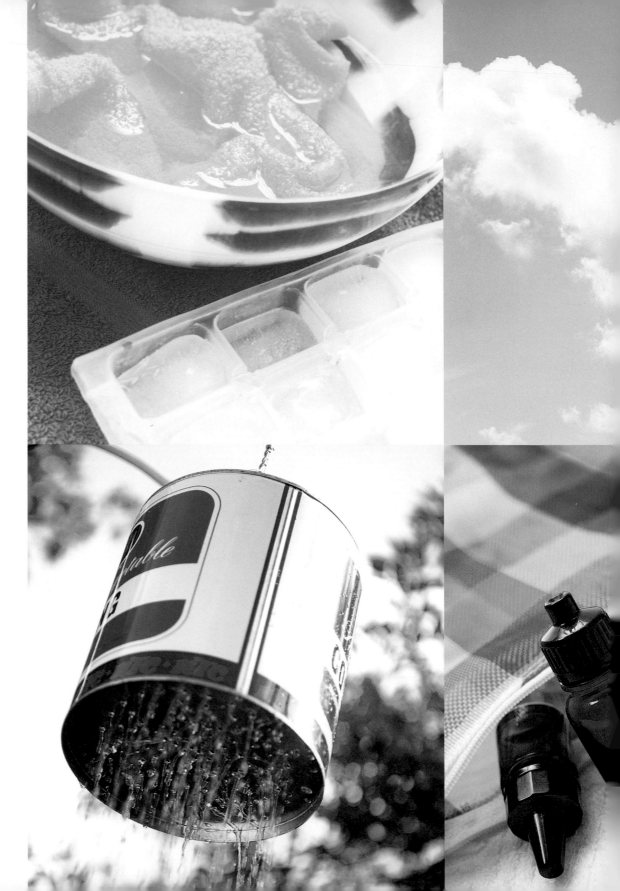

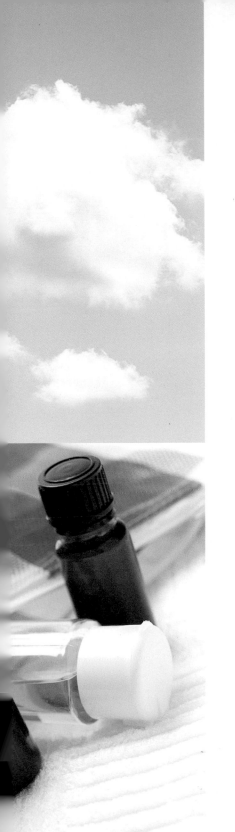

Exercise stimulates the release of neurochemicals that have a naturally uplifting, painkilling effect. It increases the metabolic rate, which helps maintain a healthy weight, and stimulates the flow of blood and lymph, making the release of toxins more efficient. Posture and muscle tone improve, so you feel fitter and healthier. It also provides a change of focus, which breaks the concentration from work or other matters causing anxiety.

When your objective is to enhance your quality of life by improving your ability to relax, exercise can take many forms and need not be a physically punishing regime. Whatever you choose, though, needs to be fulfilling and rewarding to you so

exercise for a clear mind

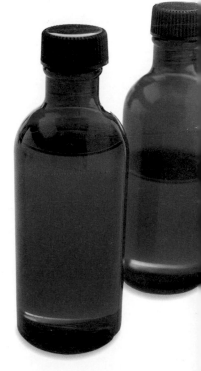

you maintain the regularity. Any exercise you enjoy will aid relaxation, but don't overdo it if you are feeling exhausted. Swimming is effective if you need to build up fitness carefully, since water is gently supportive and goes hand in hand with relaxation. Fresh air can be deeply relaxing, so anything like golf, riding, tennis, or football will help you relax and breathe deeply, releasing the day's tensions. Some of the ancient forms of exercise which incorporate stretching with deep breathing exercises and relaxation, such as tai chi and yoga, are profoundly effective, while meditation helps attune awareness and brings mental processes under voluntary control. Stress-related conditions respond extremely well to these practices, as they help quieten the mind and let you access your inner strength.

35

Many of us exclude our own needs for the sake of others and fail to appreciate the long-term costs of this to our health and quality of life. Book time for yourself as you would make appointments at work, so they are built into your routine. Don't regard this as selfish, consider what those who rely on you would do if you became ill. Making time to pamper yourself is an essential aspect of maintaining your perspective on life and your ability to relax. A few sessions a month doing something indulgent can make all the difference. We all need something to look forward to, whether it is an aromatherapy massage or beauty treatment, or an afternoon spent in a health spa.

Jacuzzis are wonderfully relaxing, but bear in mind that communal spas are a cocktail of antiseptic chemicals and bacteria, so they are not the things to use if your immune system is compromised. Many baths are equipped with Jacuzzi modifications, and there are also fittings available that can be placed in the bottom of the tub to create a jet of bubbles. The warm, circulating water makes the use of essential oils particularly appropriate, as it aids vaporization. (*See* Bath blends on p. 45, but add only one drop of each oil and repeat after 15 minutes, with the exception of benzoin.)

A sauna followed by a cool shower stimulates the circulation and helps ease tension in the shoulders and back, but don't stay in too long since it can leave you feeling drained. Detoxifying essences are often added to the water poured on the coals, but to encourage deep relaxation add orange, mandarin, bergamot, or lavender essence. Drink plenty of water during and after the sauna to avoid dehydration and assist detoxification.

Deeply relaxing steam rooms also have a detoxifying effect and can be less harsh than the dry heat of saunas. A cool shower afterward will make your skin tingle and your muscles relax. The use of essential oils will be at the discretion of the operator, but you could place a small bowl of water with a few drops of essence next to the steam vents; as the steam is released, the oils will vaporize. Try petitgrain, lavender, or camomile.

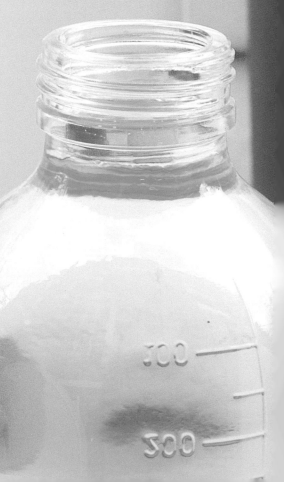

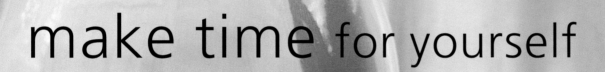

make time for yourself

Pampering treats will help to relax the body and do wonders for the mind and spirit.

An aromatherapy massage is one of the ultimate ways to unwind, since the relaxing vapors are inhaled and the essences are absorbed as the physical action eases muscular tension. Pay special attention to areas where tension builds up— the face, head, neck, shoulders, back, and feet—and concentrate on where the muscles look tense and rigid. Massage techniques can be learnt from step-by-step books or videos, including self-massage, which is particularly effective on the feet and hands where there are reflex points relating to other areas of the body. Warm the oil and your hands first, and keep your back straight while giving a massage. Never apply pressure on the spine itself; work on each side of it. Apply pressure moving toward the heart to assist the weaker blood flow as it returns to the heart via the veins. Do not apply downward pressure and glide the hands gently, avoiding sudden, uneven movements.

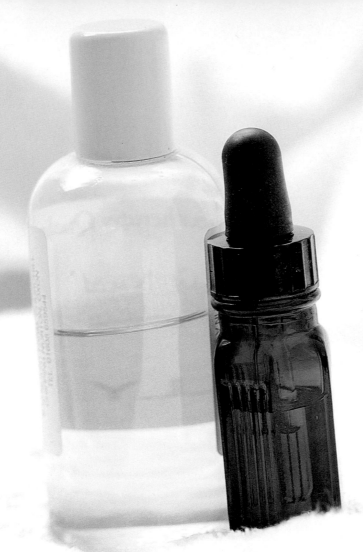

easing tension

The back and shoulders are easy places to gain a smooth, fluid rhythm and often hold a great deal of tension; after a massage the back will often look and feel totally different. Your partner should lie face down, and you can kneel astride them or at their side. Start by working from the base of the spine up, applying gentle, flowing pressure, making fanning motions with your hands flat. Repeat before concentrating on the upper shoulders, alternately squeezing and releasing, kneading the muscles on each side of the neck. Use very gentle pressure at the start, and increase it gradually as the muscles begin to relax. When the shoulders are more relaxed, turn your partner's head to the other side and slide your thumbs down each side of the spine from the nape of the neck to the base. To help release tension in the lower back, use small, gentle, circular or rotating movements with the thumbs. Pay particular attention to any areas of the back where the muscles are bunched up or tight to touch. Gently knead the area and then create friction by quickly moving your palms backward and forward over the area, building up the heat to make the muscles relax more rapidly. Use long, flowing effleurage movements, sliding your palms down the back on each side of the spine and lightly pulling them up again. Finish by softly stroking your fingers along the spine.

The neck is an area where tension builds, often flowing up from the shoulders and causing anything from minor discomfort and tension headaches to chronic pain and restriction of movement. With your partner on their back, slide your hand behind their neck and gently squeeze, pressing and releasing your fingers first on one side and then on the other. Slide the tips of the fingers of both hands down to the base of the neck and gently pull the muscles up toward the cranium. Do this several times using firm but gentle pressure. Finally, release tension at the base of the cranium with rotating movements made by the fingertips.

The head and face often hold a great deal of tension, particularly in the forehead and the base of the head where the neck joins the cranium. Massage the scalp with your fingertips in a rotating motion as if you were washing the hair, applying firm pressure to release tension. Facial skin is very delicate and should be massaged very gently. Use a small amount of oil blend and make sure it doesn't go near the eyes. Release lines of tension in the forehead by pulling your thumbs gently but firmly from the middle of the forehead across to the temples. Repeat several times. Then stroke the thumbs from one side of the head to the other, starting on one side near the temples, moving up toward the hairline from the brow. Place the fingertips on the temples and use gentle circular movements to relieve tension headaches and the buildup of pressure. Gently stroke the thumbs across the cheekbones, working from the center of the face over the rest of the cheeks, drawing the skin gently toward the hairline.

The feet are assumed to be ticklish, but a firm massage can be supremely relaxing. Apply firm pressure across the sole of the foot with your thumbs, paying particular attention to the instep —the spinal zone in reflexology. Gently pull each toe, then place your thumb firmly over the center of the instep so the thumb pad presses under the center of the ball of the foot. This relates to the solar plexus, the emotional center in reflexology.

base oils for blending

A full-body massage will use up approximately 2 tablespoons of base oil. If you prefer, mix 4 ounces at a time and store it in a cool, dark place. *See* pp. 14–15 for the principles of blending.

Apricot kernel oil An expensive, virtually clear oil, rich in vitamins, minerals, and proteins. It is useful for facial preparations, as it is light and soothing. Use up to 100 percent dilution.

Avocado oil The dark green oil is rich in vitamins, minerals, and essential fatty acids. It is helpful for dehydrated and mature skin, eczema, and psoriasis. Use at 5–25 percent dilution.

Evening primrose oil A pale yellow oil rich in vitamins, minerals, and GLA (Gamma Linolenic Acid). It is helpful for aging skin, eczema, and psoriasis. Use up to 100 percent dilution.

Grape seed oil The very pale green oil contains vitamins, minerals, and proteins. It is good for all skin types; the light oil is gently emollient and leaves skin silky and smooth, but not greasy. Use up to 100 percent dilution.

Hempseed oil A moisturizing brown-green oil that has a soothing effect on muscular tension, even before the addition of essential oils. Use on its own or in combination with another base oil.

Jojoba oil Strictly a wax, not an oil, which is pale yellow and makes a luxurious, sensual addition to blends. It is soothing and balancing for oily and dry skin, eczema, and psoriasis, and helpful for arthritis. Use at 5–15 percent dilution.

Olive oil The virgin cold-pressed oil is a rich dark green and contains high levels of vitamins, minerals, proteins, and essential fatty acids. It is soothing and nourishing for dry skin and related conditions. Use at 10 percent dilution.

St John's wort A red herbal tincture, helpful for sore muscles, neck and back pain, inflamed skin, oily hair and skin, and nervous conditions. Do not use before exposure to the sun, since it is phototoxic. Use at 10–50 percent dilution.

Sweet almond oil The pale yellow oil is rich in vitamins, minerals, and proteins. It is suitable for all skin types, especially irritated, dry, or sore skin. Use up to 100 percent dilution.

Wheat germ oil Do not use if you have gluten allergies. A yellow oil rich in vitamins, minerals, and proteins, helpful for dry or aging skin, eczema, and psoriasis. Its antioxidant properties prolong the life of blends. Use at 5–15 percent dilution.

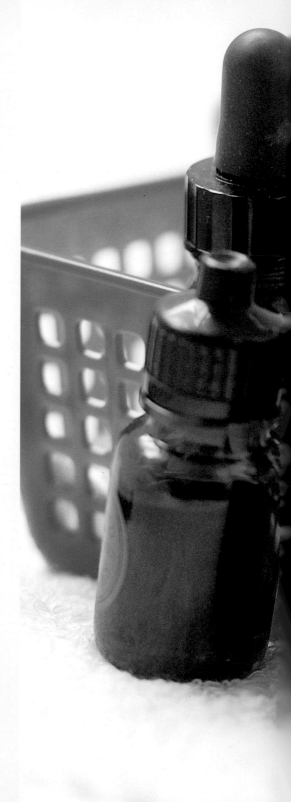

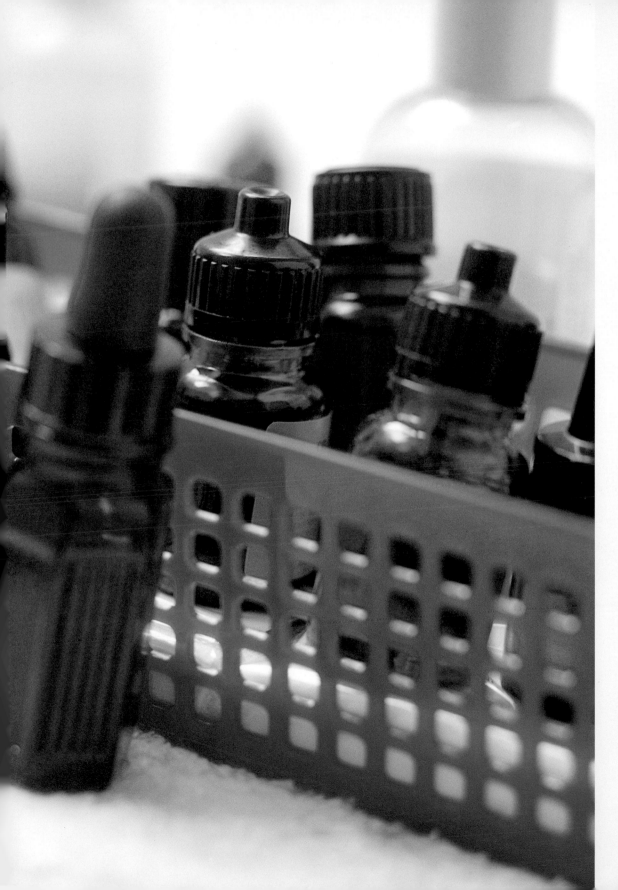

massage oils

Blends for moderate stress

Add one of the following blends to 2 tablespoons of sweet almond oil:

Lavender essence, 5 drops

Orange essence, 3 drops

Petitgrain essence, 2 drops

Bergamot essence, 5 drops

Geranium essence, 3 drops

Ylang ylang essence, 2 drops

Orange essence, 4 drops

Sandalwood essence, 4 drops

Benzoin essence, 1 drop

Blends for chronic stress

Mix 1 ounce of sweet almond oil and 1 teaspoon of hempseed oil or St John's wort, then add one of the following blends:

Lavender essence, 6 drops

Clary sage essence, 3 drops

Frankincense essence, 3 drops

Geranium essence, 5 drops

Ylang ylang essence, 4 drops

Vetiver essence, 1 drop

Bergamot essence, 5 drops

Petitgrain essence, 4 drops

Neroli essence, 1 drop

Bergamot essence, 5 drops

Sandalwood essence, 4 drops

Rose essence, 1 drop

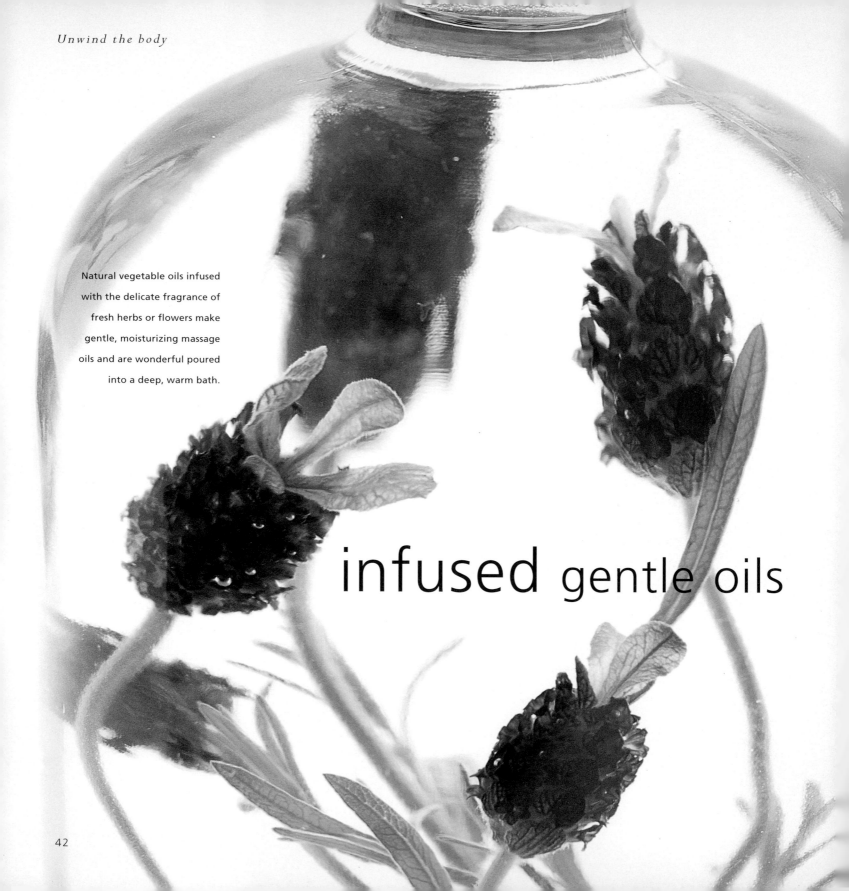

Natural vegetable oils infused
with the delicate fragrance of
fresh herbs or flowers make
gentle, moisturizing massage
oils and are wonderful poured
into a deep, warm bath.

infused gentle oils

This is one of the most ancient, simple, and inexpensive methods of making gentle, fragrant massage or bath oils using herbs and flowers from the garden. These oils can even be used in cooking, and they make lovely gifts.

For a relaxing infusion, use herbs such as marjoram, lavender, camomile, or clary sage. Fragile flowers like roses can also be used, although the woody herbs seem to infuse most effectively. Use a bland vegetable oil such as sweet almond, grape seed, or apricot kernel.

Wash the fresh herbs or flower petals with warm water and let them dry. Then, use boiling water to sterilize a wide-necked jar with a tight-fitting lid and also let it dry. Fill the jar ¼–⅓ full with the plant material and slowly pour the vegetable oil over it, gently shaking the jar as you do so to release trapped air bubbles. Pour the oil right to the top to make sure there is no air trapped in the jar, since this would speed up the oxidation process and turn the mixture cloudy and rancid. Seal the jar and place it in a warm place—on a sunny windowsill, or near a furnace or radiator. When all the plant material has lost its color, remove it from the jar and replace it with more clean, fresh herbs, flowers, or petals. Repeat this process two to four more times depending on the required strength of the aroma and therapeutic effect. When the mixture is ready, take out all the plant material and strain the oil through a fine filter to remove any remaining plant particles or sediment. Pour the pure aromatic oil into a sterile, airtight container and store it in a dark, cool place.

Infused oils will contain many of the therapeutic and aromatic qualities of the chosen plant's essential oil, but it will not have nearly as strong an effect as the essence itself. Infused oils can also be prepared by gently heating the vegetable oil and plant material to speed up the process, but the resulting product is of inferior quality.

Many of us shower instead of making time for baths, but nothing beats a luxurious deep bath for pure relaxation. Twice a week take the time to allow yourself a real soak. It must be at a time when you will be left in peace, either early in the morning, last thing at night, or during the day—the timing is immaterial, but the quantity and quality is important. You need at least 30 minutes for sheer unadulterated relaxation.

Essential oils add a whole new dimension to the warmth and support the water offers. They generate relaxation on every level—physical, emotional, and spiritual—enhancing your ability

bathe the body; cleanse the mind

Soothing foot bath

If you truly can't make time for a bath, if you are too tired to run it, or if you need a quick-fix relaxation boost, soak your feet in a foot bath for 10 minutes. This seemingly old-fashioned remedy is a wonderfully soothing, easy way of benefiting from the combination of warm water and essential oils without having a full bath, especially if you have been on your feet all day. Use the blends in the same proportions, but half the number of drops.

to let go of worries. Some help you breathe deeply, others help reduce blood pressure, and many have an uplifting effect. In a nutshell, a bath without oils is half the experience it could be.

Always add the oils after the water has been run, or some of the essence will have evaporated before you can gain the benefits. Some relaxing essences are phototoxic, such as orange, bergamot, and mandarin, so avoid exposing your skin to direct sunlight immediately after bathing with these. Add a maximum of 10 drops of oil to your bath, but never use more than 1 drop of benzoin, which can be an irritant. For a child, the elderly, or anyone with sensitive skin, dilute the oil blend in a teaspoon of vegetable oil or milk to fully disperse the molecules.

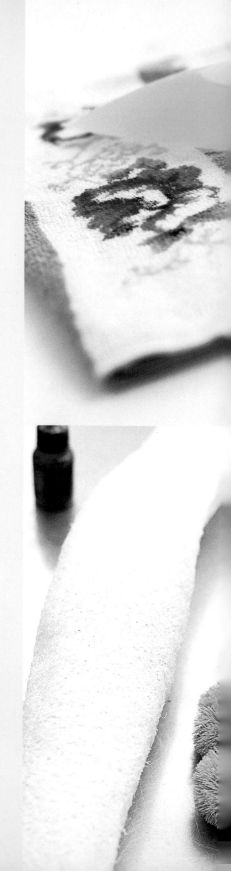

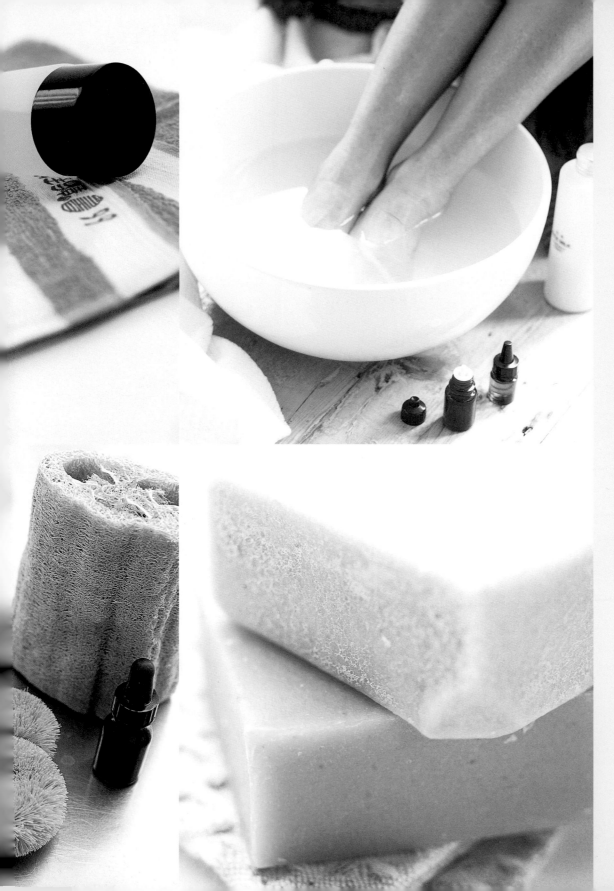

bath blends

Add one of the following blends to a full bathtub, or double the number of drops and add the essential oils to 4 ounces of bland shower gel or bubble bath base; shake well before use:

Blends for moderate stress

Lavender essence, 5 drops

Orange essence, 3 drops

Petitgrain essence, 2 drops

Bergamot essence, 5 drops

Geranium essence, 3 drops

Ylang ylang essence, 2 drops

Orange essence, 4 drops

Sandalwood essence, 4 drops

Benzoin essence, 1 drop

Blends for chronic stress

Lavender essence, 6 drops

Clary sage essence, 3 drops

Frankincense essence, 3 drops

Geranium essence, 5 drops

Ylang ylang essence, 4 drops

Vetiver essence, 1 drop

Bergamot essence, 5 drops

Petitgrain essence, 4 drops

Neroli essence, 1 drop

Bergamot essence, 5 drops

Sandalwood essence, 4 drops

Rose essence, 1 drop

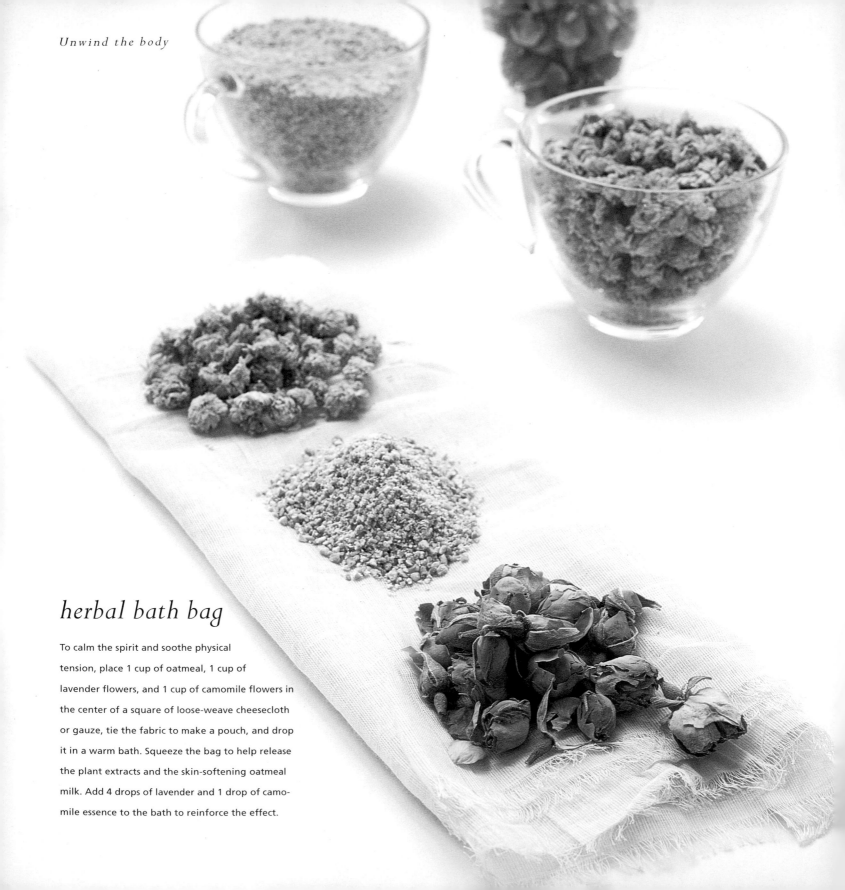

herbal bath bag

To calm the spirit and soothe physical
tension, place 1 cup of oatmeal, 1 cup of
lavender flowers, and 1 cup of camomile flowers in
the center of a square of loose-weave cheesecloth
or gauze, tie the fabric to make a pouch, and drop
it in a warm bath. Squeeze the bag to help release
the plant extracts and the skin-softening oatmeal
milk. Add 4 drops of lavender and 1 drop of camomile essence to the bath to reinforce the effect.

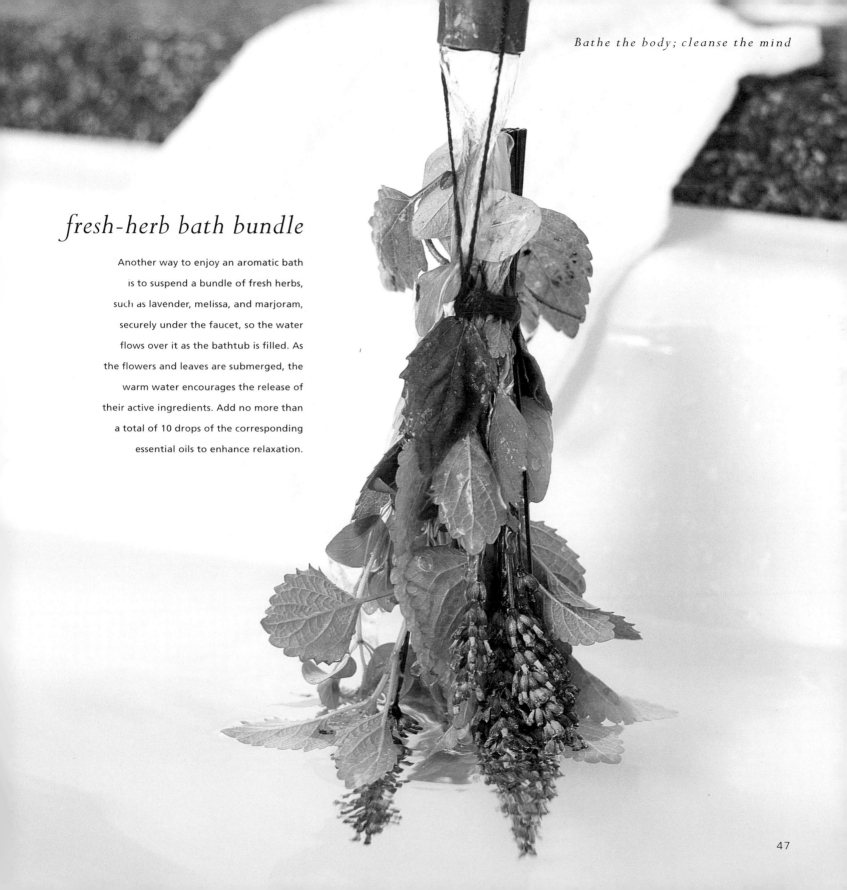

fresh-herb bath bundle

Another way to enjoy an aromatic bath
is to suspend a bundle of fresh herbs,
such as lavender, melissa, and marjoram,
securely under the faucet, so the water
flows over it as the bathtub is filled. As
the flowers and leaves are submerged, the
warm water encourages the release of
their active ingredients. Add no more than
a total of 10 drops of the corresponding
essential oils to enhance relaxation.

47

Unwind the body

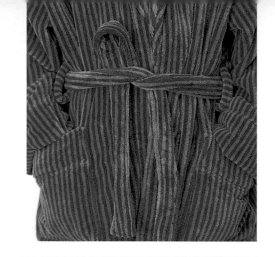

A relaxing bath last thing before bed is the perfect way to unwind after a busy day. Use sedative essences that will calm your mind and leave your skin soft and fragrant. Dry yourself gently with a large, soft towel, then wrap yourself in a luxurious robe.

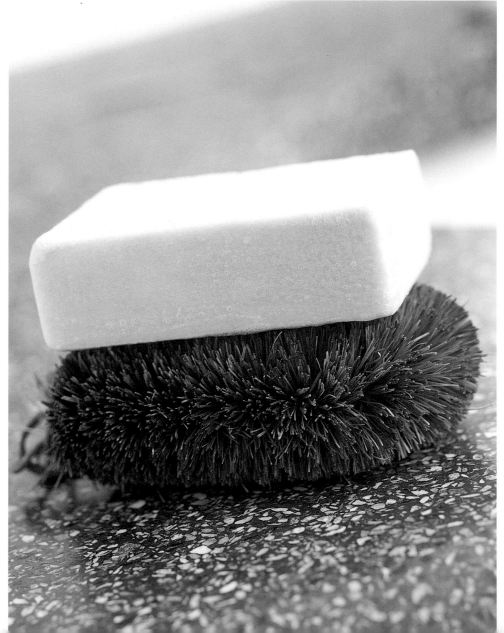

Bedtime bathing

To encourage a sound and restful sleep that will help rejuvenate your body and mind, have a long soak in a deep, warm bath using a blend that includes some of the most sedative essential oils, such as camomile, marjoram, or lavender. Do not have the water too hot, since it will leave you feeling drained rather than pleasantly relaxed. Dim the lights or fill the room with candles for a magical, supremely soothing atmosphere.

Turn the experience into a ritual that really lets you wind down, making it as enjoyable and indulgent as possible. Take the opportunity to reflect on the day and consciously put all your worries to the back of your mind. Drink a cup of calming camomile tea or soothing hot milk—whatever helps you relax. All the time, breathe deeply and steadily so you fully inhale the therapeutic vapors and release the tension in your chest and stomach muscles. After soaking for at least 30 minutes, get out slowly and gently dab yourself dry, do not rub vigorously. Then wrap yourself in a warm bathrobe before sinking into bed.

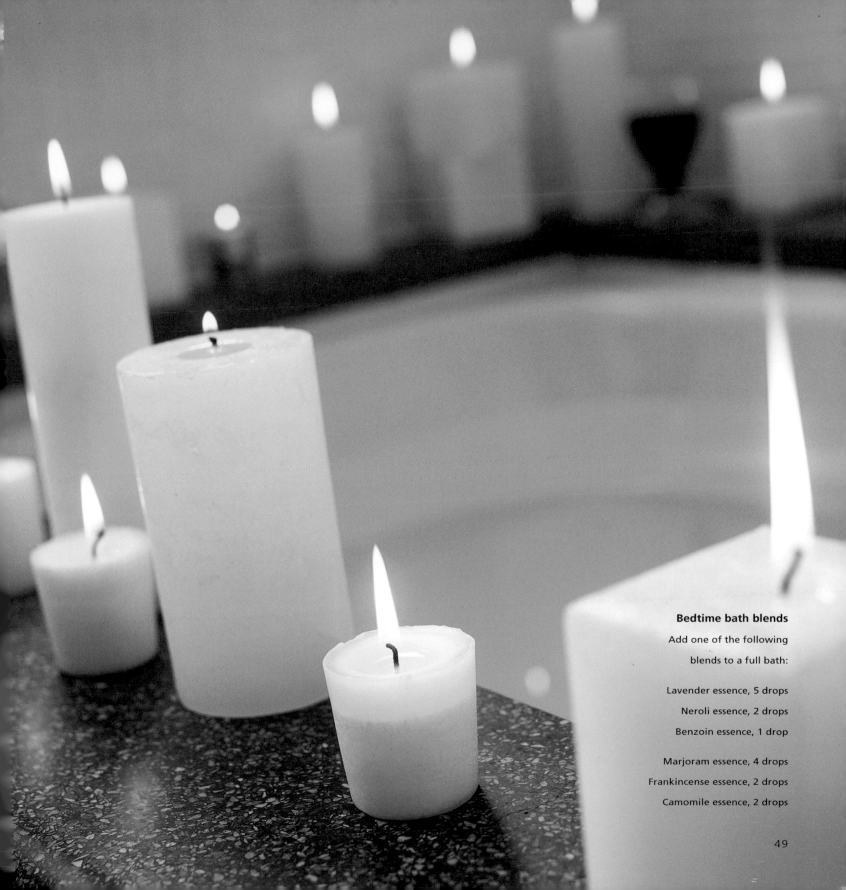

Bedtime bath blends

Add one of the following
blends to a full bath:

Lavender essence, 5 drops
Neroli essence, 2 drops
Benzoin essence, 1 drop

Marjoram essence, 4 drops
Frankincense essence, 2 drops
Camomile essence, 2 drops

moisturizing body oils & creams

Moisturizing body balm

1 ounce yellow, unrefined beeswax

4 ounces sweet almond oil

4 ounces orange-flower water

One of the blends of essences

Shave the beeswax into a glass or ceramic bowl and add the sweet almond oil. Place the bowl in a saucepan of water and heat it gently until the beeswax has melted. Meanwhile, heat the orange-flower water in another double boiler. When both the oil mixture and the flower water are warm, remove them from the heat and combine them. Add the drops of essential oil and stir them in well, then pour the balm into an airtight glass jar and refrigerate.

Body oil for normal skin

Mix 1 ounce sweet almond oil

1 teaspoon avocado oil

or wheat germ oil

2 teaspoons evening primrose oil

2 teaspoons jojoba oil, then add

one of the blends of essences.

Body oil for dry skin

Mix 2 ounces sweet almond oil

1 teaspoon jojoba oil

1 teaspoon avocado oil, then add

one of the blends of essences.

Body lotion or cream

Add either of the blends of essences to 2 tablespoons of a natural body lotion or cream.

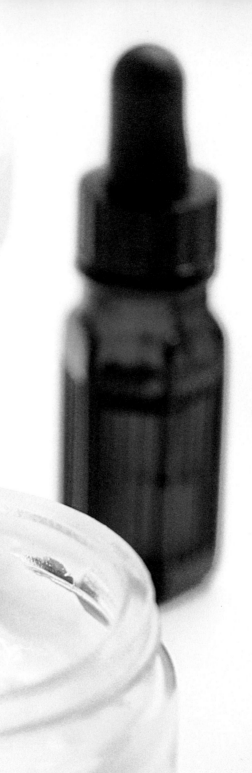

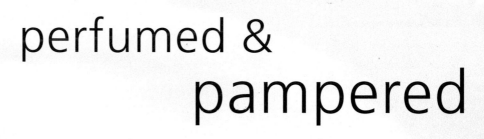

perfumed &
pampered

Daytime blend of essences

An uplifting blend to promote a
positive, calm outlook to the day:

Geranium essence, 6 drops

Frankincense essence, 4 drops

Rose essence, 2 drops

Bedtime blend of essences

A supremely relaxing blend to
encourage a peaceful sleep:

Lavender essence, 10 drops

Camomile essence, 2 drops

Neroli essence, 2 drops

Moisturizing creams, lotions, and oils are ideal mediums for
applying essential oils to the body, and pampering the skin
with wonderfully scented, nourishing preparations can be
extremely relaxing. Blends of essences incorporated into
beauty treatments enhance skin condition and texture, and
aid the elimination of toxins by stimulating the circulation.
In addition to being such a pleasure to use and leaving the skin
subtly fragrant, the soothing, tranquilizing action of the
essences relaxes the muscles and soothes the emotions.

Essential oils work on the skin in many ways to keep it
healthy, promoting good circulation, detoxification, cell
renewal and regeneration, and maintaining a balanced output of
sebum (the skin's natural oil). The body oils contain nutritive,
emollient vegetable oils that have rich, regenerative properties,
but if you prefer a less greasy texture, add the blends to natural
purchased or homemade lotions or creams. Use these beauty
treatments every day to perfume your skin and keep it in peak
condition, applying them after bathing to increase absorption.
Mix fairly small amounts of body oil or balm at a time, so the
essences are fresh and have maximum therapeutic effect.

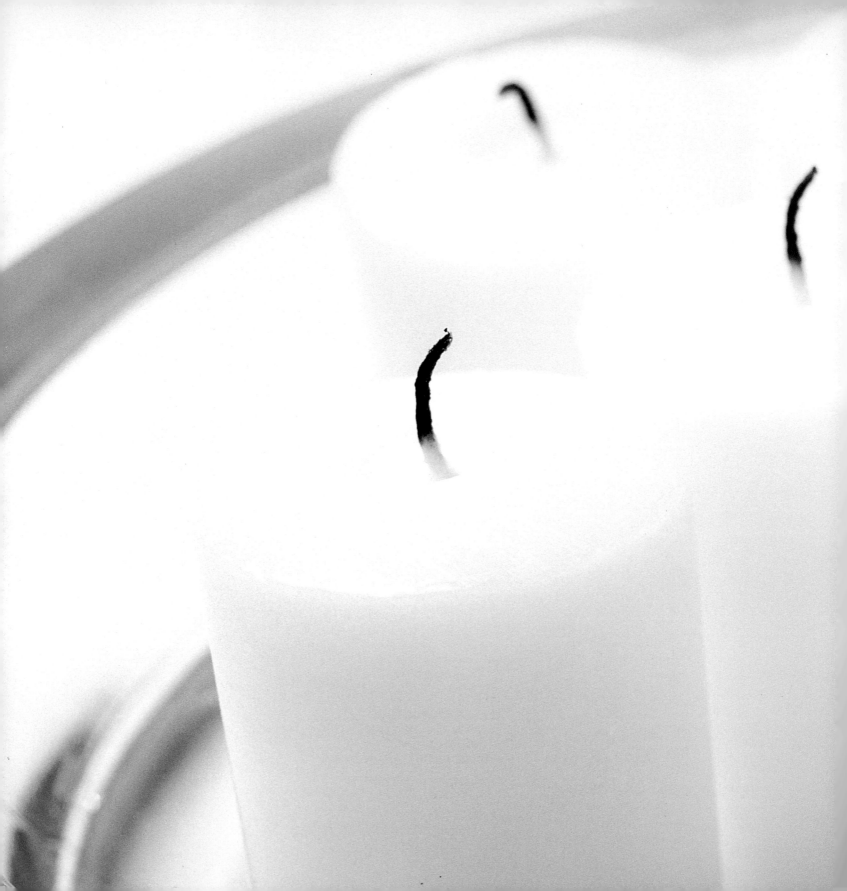

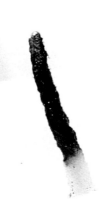

Use mood-enhancing blends of
essential oils to fill the air around
you with a wonderfully relaxing
perfume that will create a tranquil,
calming, and restful atmosphere.

peaceful
SURROUNDINGS

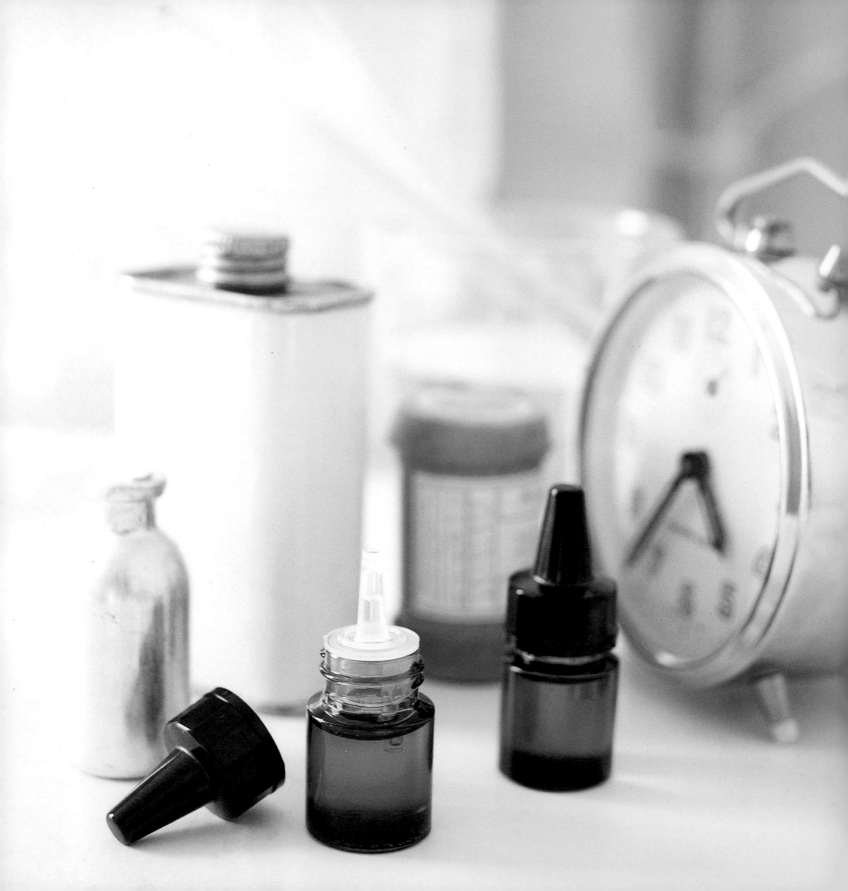

It is impossible to relax physically if we can't switch off mentally, and impossible to think productively if our minds are full of anxiety. Essential oils have a unique balancing effect on the emotions, and filling your home or work space with soothing aromas will help create a tranquil atmosphere and leave your surroundings gorgeously fragrant. Essential oils are endlessly

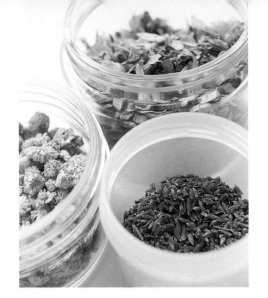

relaxing fragrances for

a mellow mood

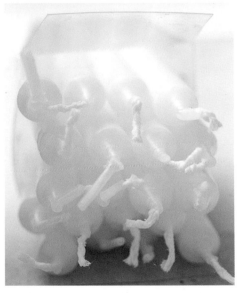

versatile: they can be vaporized; added to humidifiers, diffusers, or melted candle wax; incorporated into the wash; or added to water and dispersed using a spray. All these methods will help make the home a peaceful sanctuary to retreat to at the end of a hectic day, where you can relax, unwind, and restore your spirits.

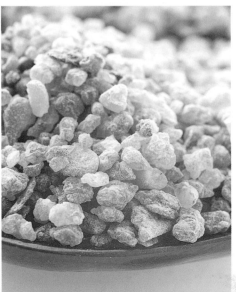

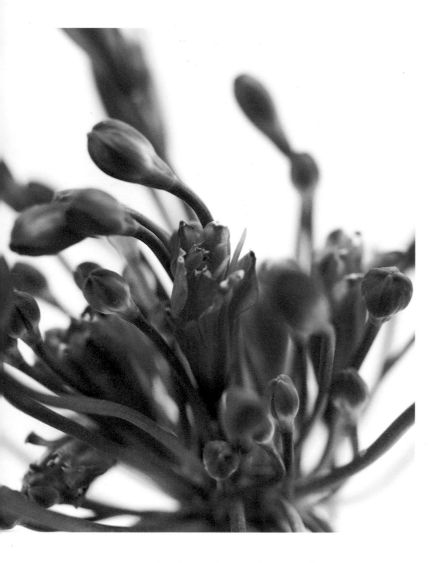

The scent of a room makes an immediate impression as soon as you enter and reflects the people who use it and their way of life. There are endless ways to fill your home with a wonderful fragrance that greets you as you open the door—whether it is the freshness of laundry, the warm aromas of baking, the comforting scent of newly waxed wood, or the heady perfume of flowers.

One of the simplest, most versatile ways to scent the home is with uplifting, harmonizing essential oils. There are many ways to release them into the air, and whatever medium you choose, you can use different blends depending on the room, time of day, and mood you wish to inspire. Vaporizers are perhaps the most usual way of dispersing essential oil molecules. Traditional models include a ceramic bowl, which holds water and a few drops of essence, balanced on a hollow base that houses a small candle. The candle heats the water so the volatile essential oil molecules are vaporized and gradually released into the air. Electric models have an indentation to hold the essences with or without a little water; unlike the candle models, these can be left unattended, but should be switched off when the oil has evaporated. Electric diffusers or humidifiers are other safe and effective ways of dispersing essences, as are bowls that can be attached to a radiator, which hold water and essential oil.

Cut flowers add life and color to any environment, and being aware of their medicinal attributes brings an added bonus. Rose essence is a potent antidepressant, and garden roses, with their traditional strong perfume, create a delightful display. Herbs such as lavender, camomile, melissa, and marjoram are as attractive to look at as many flowers and foliage, and emit strongly relaxing essences when their leaves are bruised.

subtle, floral, and uplifting

Lilies of the valley (*right*) have a delicate, sweet fragrance that fills the room, but many other flowers, such as agapanthus (*above*), are glorious to look at but have little or no natural perfume. If you buy flowers that don't have a strong scent of their own, add a drop of essential oil onto the petals of the flowers themselves, or add a few drops to the water in which they stand to enhance their perfume.

scents to
feed the soul

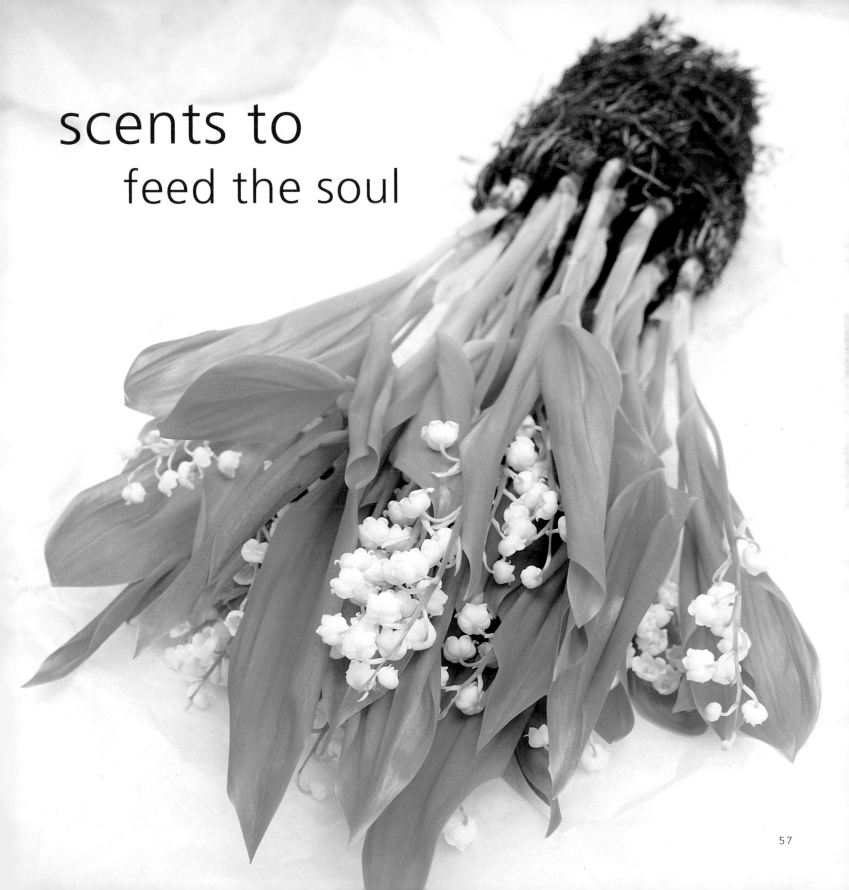

A herb garden, even if it is just a windowbox outside the kitchen window, can give endless pleasure with relatively little effort. Apart from being enjoyed for their scent and appearance, herbs can be used for cooking, baths, and potpourris.

Surrounding yourself with plants and flowers that both look beautiful and smell lovely is wonderful for the soul. Whether it is inside the house or outdoors, a touch of natural greenery and a splash of color never fail to lift the spirits.

Many people find that planting, nurturing, and watching seedlings grow is a therapeutic and satisfying process in itself, and when you choose herbs that have spiritually and physically reviving properties, every time you handle them or brush past them, you will inhale, if only in very small amounts, their natural health-giving mood-enhancing essences.

cultivate a fragrant
herb garden

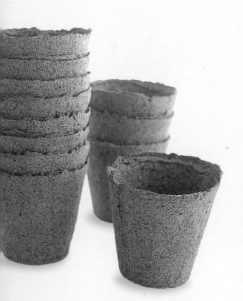

Herbs have been grown extensively since the 16th and 17th centuries for both culinary and medicinal uses, and their appeal has endured due to their simple beauty, inexpensiveness, and low maintenance. Many herbs grow well in windowboxes, and every time the window is opened the delicate fragrances waft into the room. Try growing tubs or troughs of relaxing herbs like melissa, lavender, and marjoram, all of which are as pleasing to look at as many other plants. Camomile, too, with its delicate daisylike flowers, makes a pretty ground-covering plant for an informal bed. Cuttings of homegrown herbs can be incorporated into flower displays or used in cooking; they can also be dried and used to make fragrant potpourris (*see* pp. 72–3).

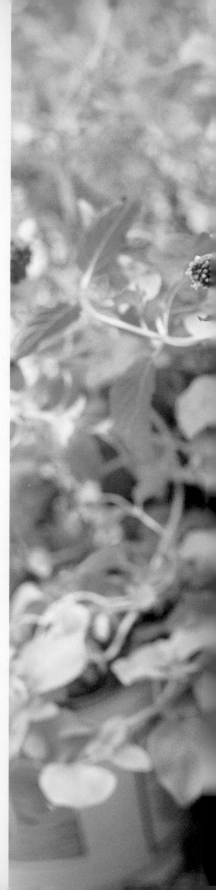

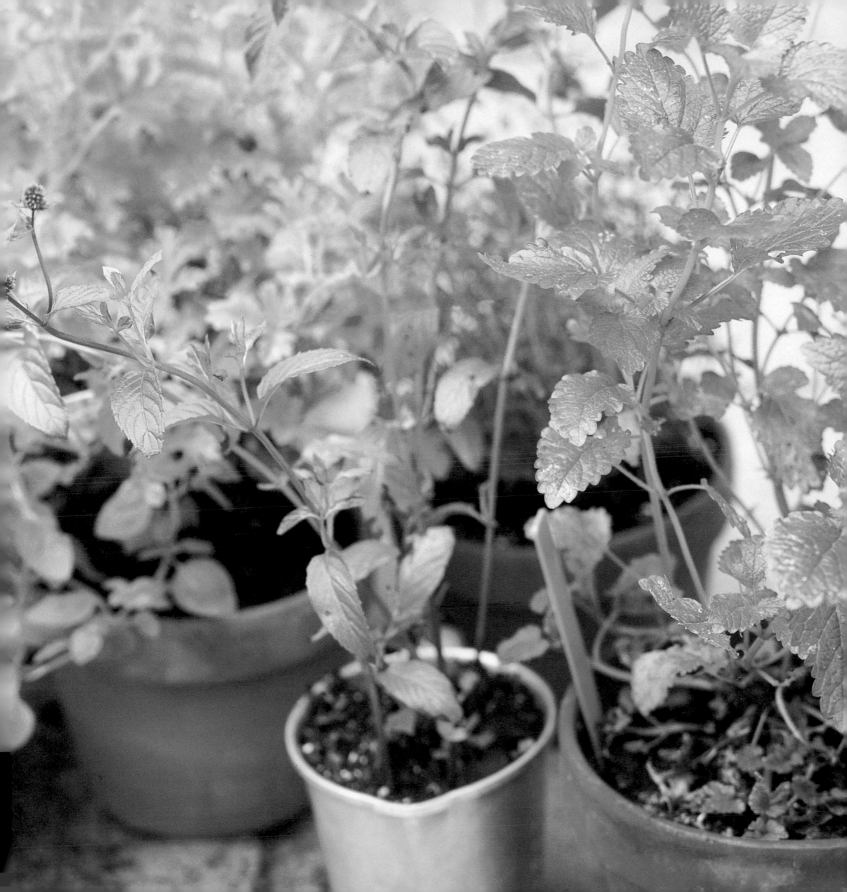

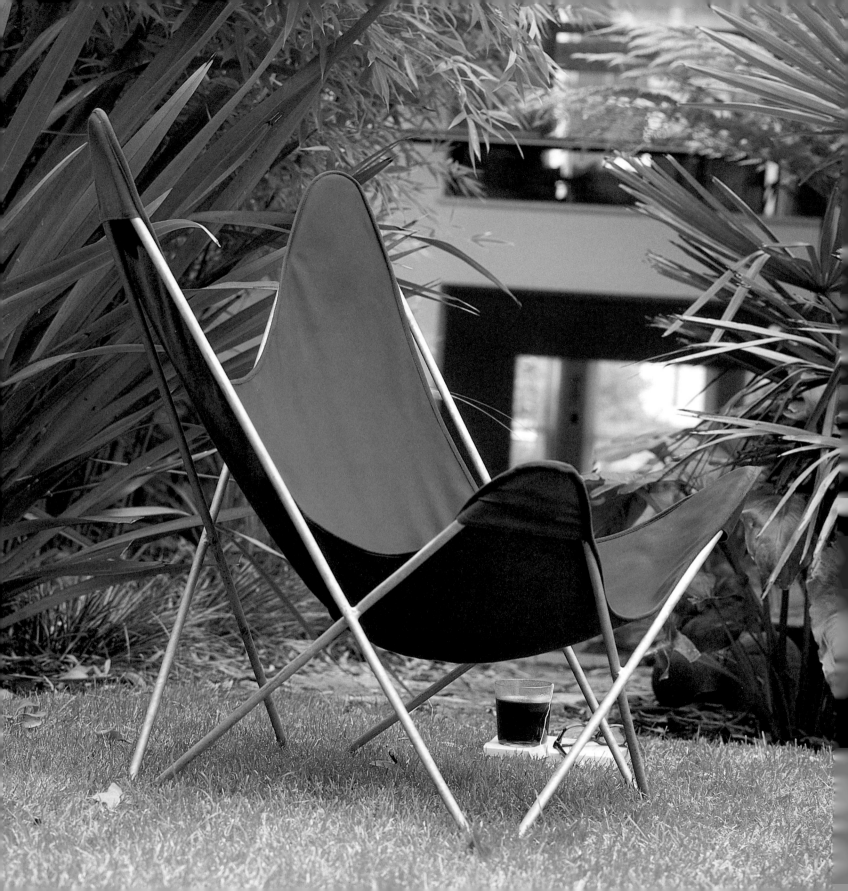

There are few more peaceful and relaxing pastimes than sitting quietly in your backyard on a warm summer's day, enjoying some simple fresh food with your family or friends, reading a good book, or just contemplating life. Even a short length of time spent in the fresh air and sunlight is uplifting and restorative for the soul, so try to allow yourself this small indulgence as often as you can. However many chores need doing, you will feel all the more efficient for taking time out for half an hour to relax in a comfortable chair in a favorite patch of lawn, enjoying a refreshing fruit or herb tea or a cooling glass of ice water. When it is too cold to sit outside for long, a brisk walk will stretch the muscles and stimulate the circulation, and a good blast of air will clear the brain and help you think clearly.

Even if you are a keen gardener, the garden should not only be a place where you work hard to create the environment you desire or the food you like to eat; it should also represent a precious opportunity for peaceful, unadulterated relaxation. Do not sit there and note all that is yet to be done; see what has been achieved and enjoy the moment.

Essential oils can be put to good use outdoors as well as in the house, since in addition to their other therapeutic and mood-enhancing properties, most of them are also repellent to insects. A ceramic vaporizer is perfect for use outdoors— it will look pretty on a terrace surrounded by terracotta flowerpots, and the candle will create a romantic ambience when daylight begins to fade. To assist relaxation, vaporize essences such as lavender, melissa, bergamot, and geranium.

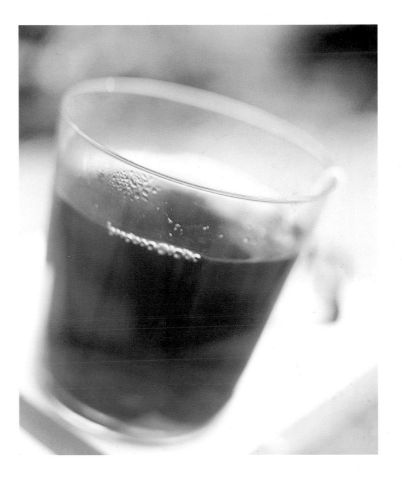

outdoor oasis

A fresh-air refuge where you can
while away a warm afternoon
provides the ideal place to rest
the body and clear the mind.

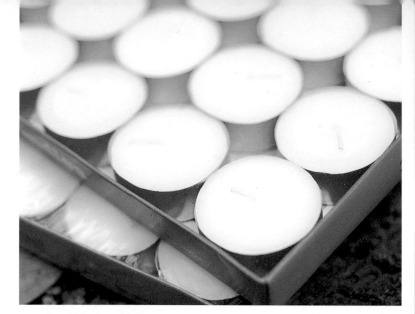

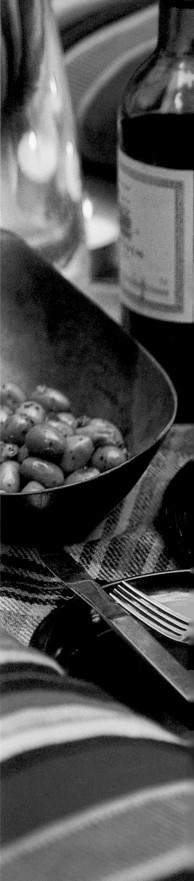

picnic at dusk

Enjoying some good food and wine in the open air, casually spread on a blanket on the ground, is possibly the most relaxed and informal way of eating on a warm evening. At dusk, light some votive candles, which look magical in the open air. When a pool of molten wax has formed around the wick, blow out the flame and carefully add a few drops of essential oil, like lavender, orange, or geranium, then relight the candle. If it is breezy, place the candles inside lanterns.

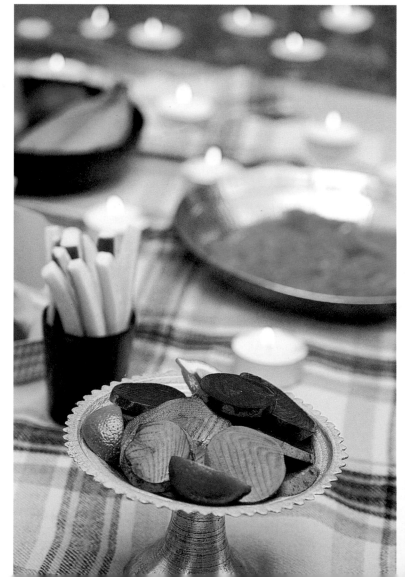

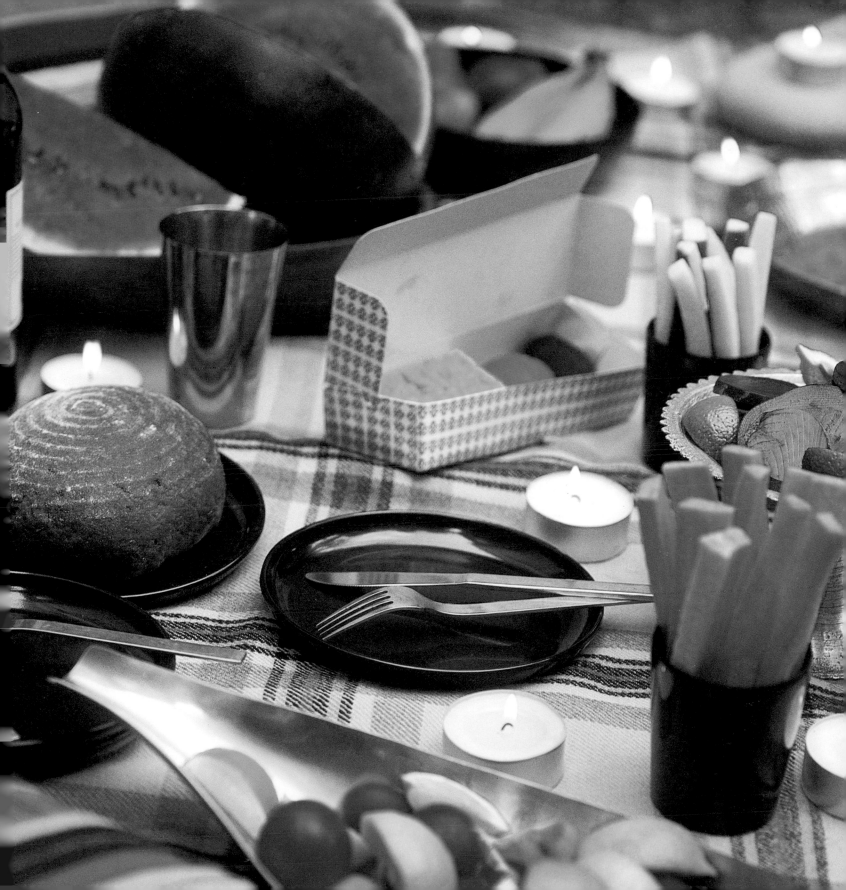

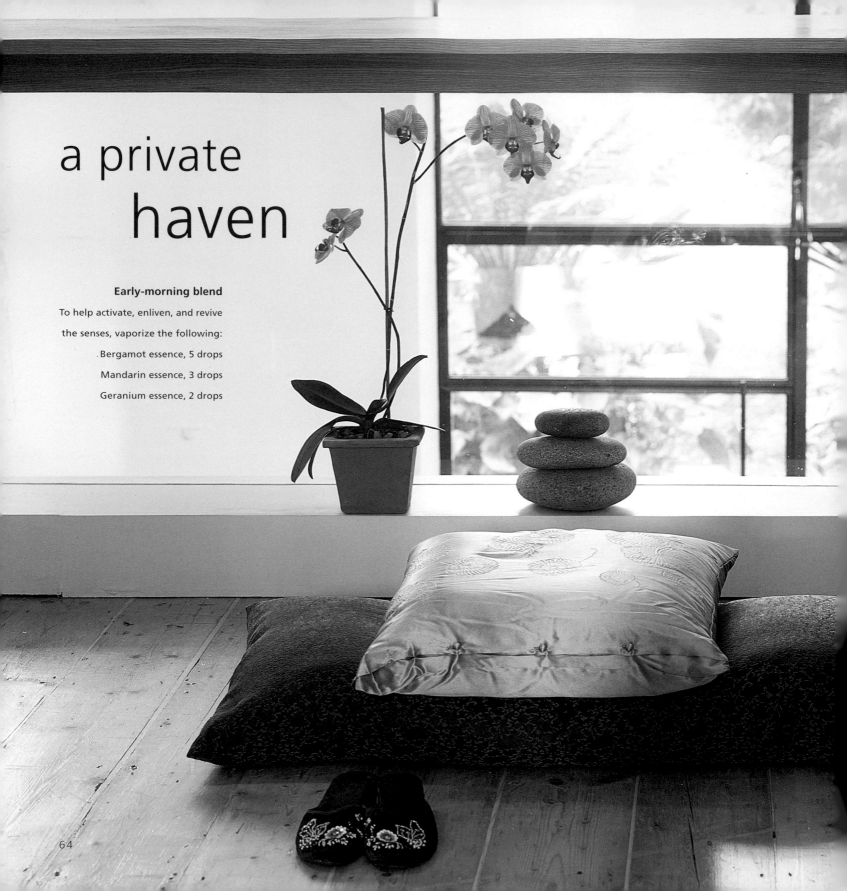

a private haven

Early-morning blend

To help activate, enliven, and revive

the senses, vaporize the following:

Bergamot essence, 5 drops

Mandarin essence, 3 drops

Geranium essence, 2 drops

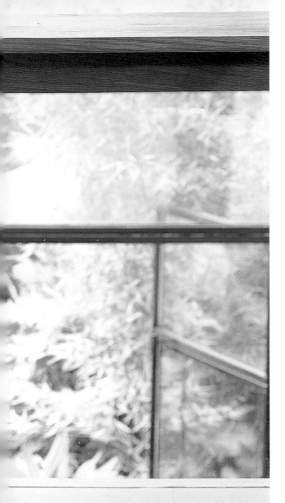

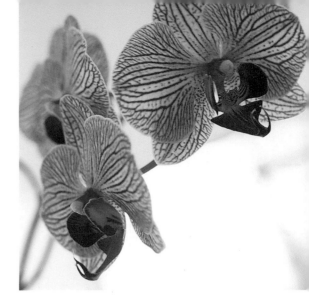

Many people who discover the benefits of yoga, meditation, or visualization, or the sheer joy of quiet contemplation, often do so in a special place that means something to them alone. This may be a favorite spot in the home or backyard, in a park, or beside a lake or the ocean. For many of us, time for ourselves is most easily found on home territory. It is a wonderful treat, therefore, to create a particular place to retreat to when time is yours. It may be a whole room or just a corner of your bedroom or living room; the point is to make it your own. The space may be clean, bare, and bright, or warm and jumbled with objects that are special to you. You might add plants or flowers and candles, or crystals to raise the energetic quality of the space.

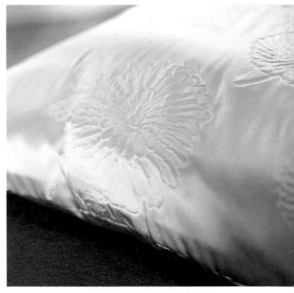

Essential oils can be put to great use to help establish a tranquil mood or assist you going into a relaxed or meditative state. To help generate a positive, optimistic outlook, spend some quiet moments in your refuge and vaporize a blend of uplifting anxiety-relieving essential oils to awaken and refresh the senses. This is your sacred place, so make it your own and enjoy it often.

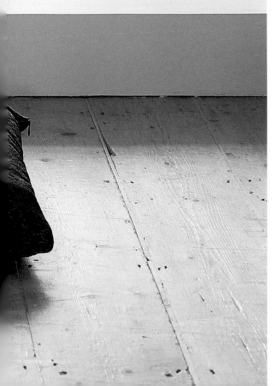

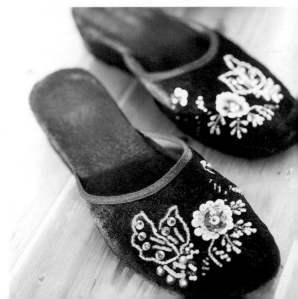

Vaporizing oils

Morning blend

To help ease the frantic pace
before lunch and release any
tension that builds up during the
morning, vaporize the following:

Orange essence, 5 drops

Petitgrain essence, 2 drops

Neroli essence, 1 drop

Afternoon blend

To help you peacefully achieve all
that is necessary before the end of
the day, vaporize the following:

Lavender essence, 5 drops

Benzoin essence, 2 drops

Rose essence, 1 drop

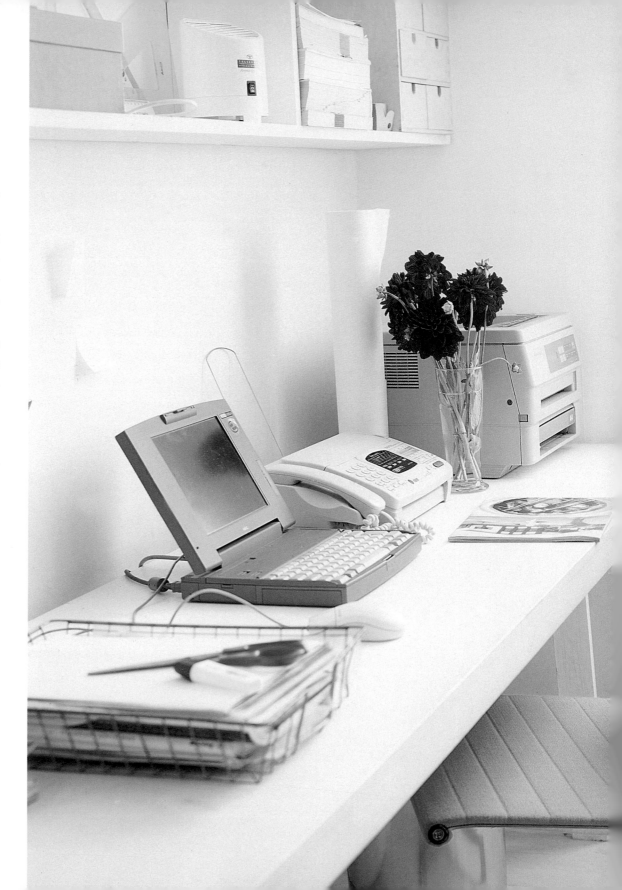

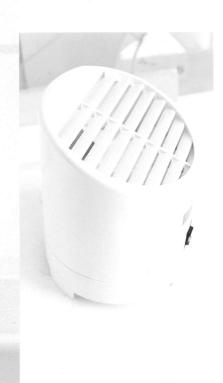

Using essential oils to relieve anxiety and stress and help promote calm feelings is nowhere more beneficial than in a work environment, where the ability to think clearly under pressure is vital. The most appropriate essences to use are ones that have a relaxing, harmonizing effect, but without a soporific action that would subdue vitality. Choose ones that have a light, refreshing aroma, like bergamot, geranium, mandarin, and orange, especially if there are other people working in the room. Bergamot and geranium, in particular, have antiseptic, antiviral properties, which will help prevent the spread of infections. Used individually or in combination, these oils will help maintain a positive, harmonious working atmosphere as well as imparting a delightful, uplifting aroma.

Easing the pressure

Electrically operated devices, such as diffusers and some humidifiers, are ideal for releasing essential oils into the work place, but make sure you buy a quiet model that won't disturb you. Diffusers, such as the one shown above, release essential oils effectively and regularly by means of an internal fan.

If you like to add natural color and life to the work place in the form of plants or cut flowers, choose those that release soothing essences, such as lavender or roses, to help promote a calm atmosphere. Inhaling from a bottle of neroli or lavender oil when you feel anxious or pressured can really boost your power to cope—and enhance your ability to unwind afterward. Lavender is also particularly useful for tension headaches; put one drop of essential oil on each index finger and massage your temples and the back of your neck, using small, firm, circular movements. Bach Flower Remedies' "Rescue Remedy" is also great for easing stress and anxiety, so keep a bottle in the office.

After a full day, not everyone is able to switch off their thoughts the moment they get into bed, however tired they are. Setting aside time to unwind fully can make all the difference. A comfortable chair to curl up in, with soft pillows to sink against, a good book to read, or peaceful music to listen to are great for clearing the mind of worries. Avoid stimulating food and drinks; a cup of herb or fruit tea is as reviving as ordinary tea or coffee, but without the stimulating effect of caffeine. Calming essential oils like frankincense, orange, and ylang ylang will help ease the pressure of the day and induce tranquility and rest. Candlelight creates a soothing atmosphere, and floating candles look magical in a glass bowl with a few drops of essence in the water or the pool of wax around the base of the wick, but extinguish the flame before adding the oils. Turkish floating candles (*bottom right*) are an unusual variation; their wicks burn in lamp oil, to which a few drops of essence can be added. Or, simply fill a bowl with hot water and add drops of essence; place it near a radiator to keep it warm, and agitate the water to disperse the essential oil molecules.

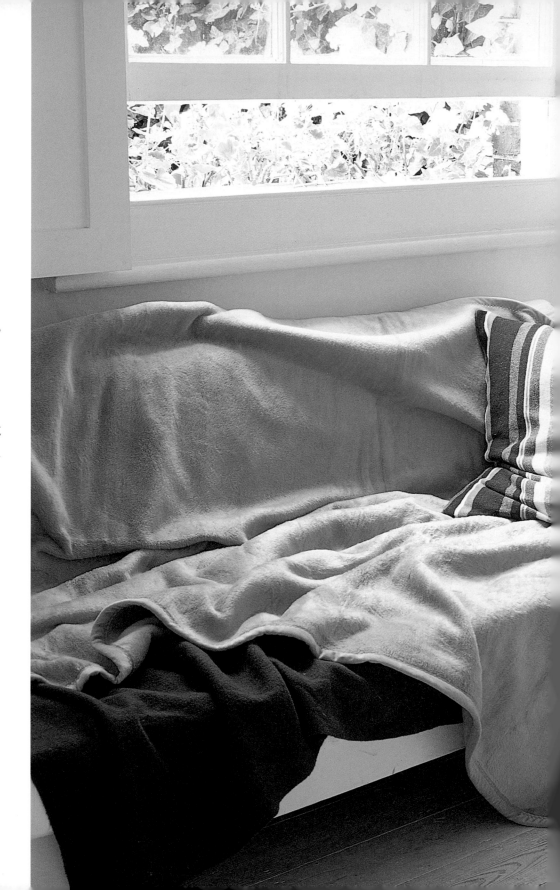

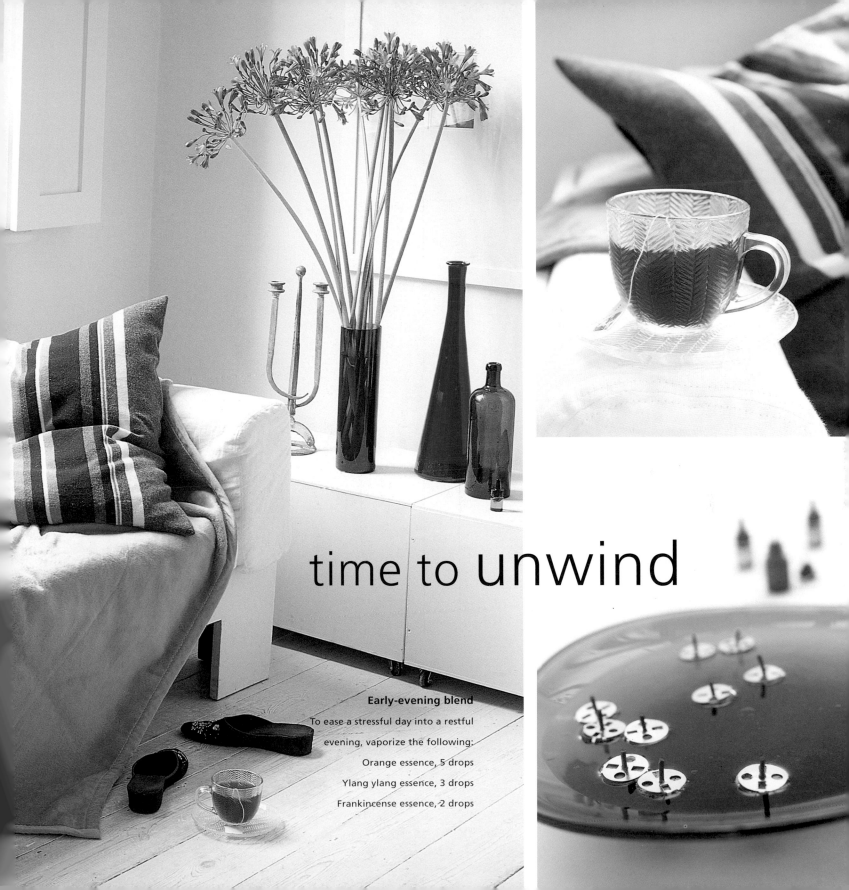

time to unwind

Early-evening blend

To ease a stressful day into a restful

evening, vaporize the following:

Orange essence, 5 drops

Ylang ylang essence, 3 drops

Frankincense essence, 2 drops

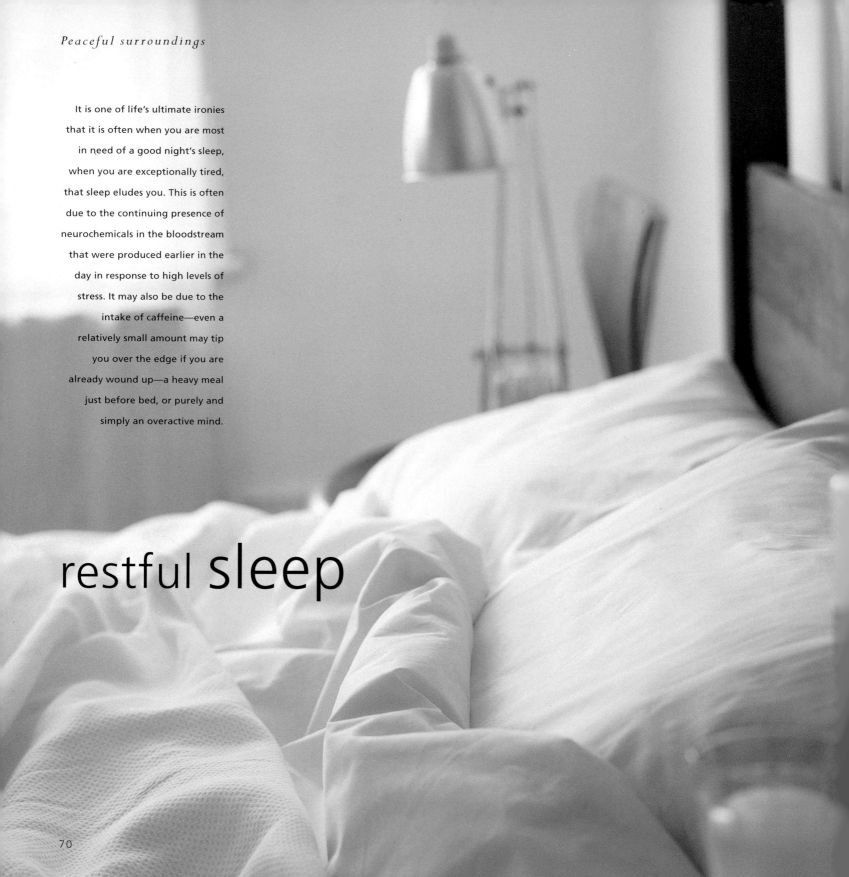

It is one of life's ultimate ironies that it is often when you are most in need of a good night's sleep, when you are exceptionally tired, that sleep eludes you. This is often due to the continuing presence of neurochemicals in the bloodstream that were produced earlier in the day in response to high levels of stress. It may also be due to the intake of caffeine—even a relatively small amount may tip you over the edge if you are already wound up—a heavy meal just before bed, or purely and simply an overactive mind.

restful sleep

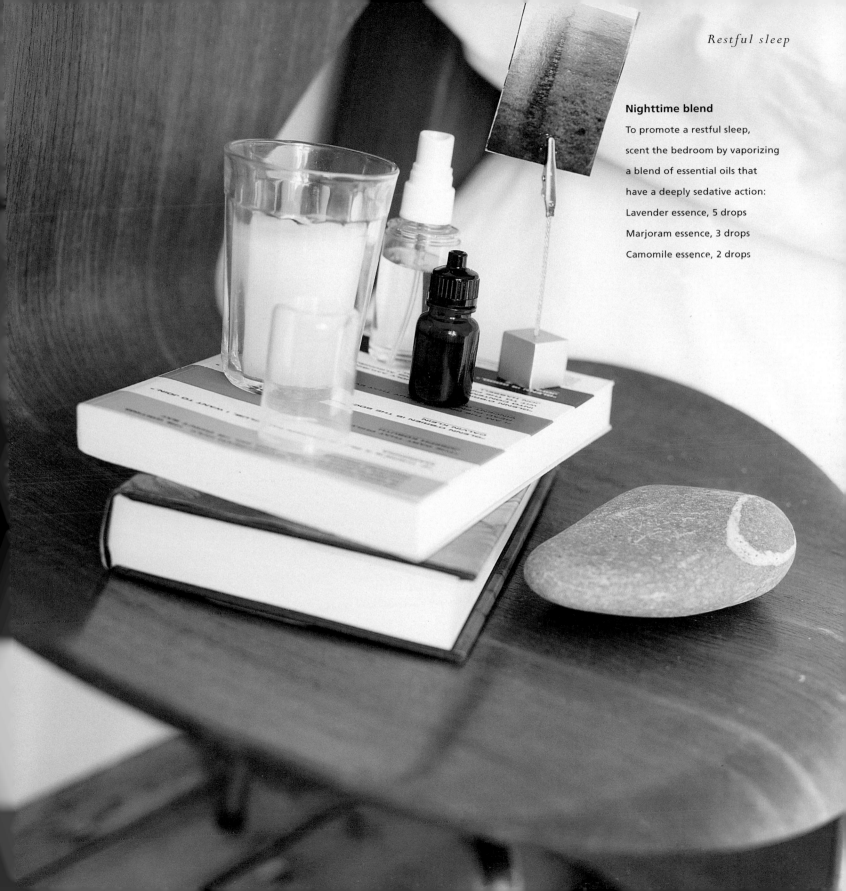

Nighttime blend

To promote a restful sleep,
scent the bedroom by vaporizing
a blend of essential oils that
have a deeply sedative action:

Lavender essence, 5 drops

Marjoram essence, 3 drops

Camomile essence, 2 drops

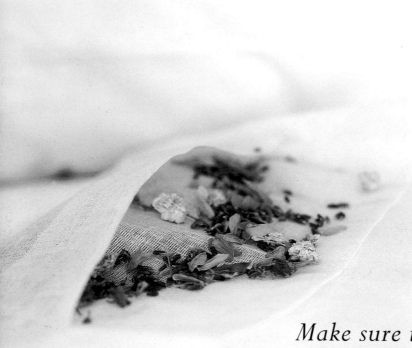

Fill your bedroom with the most relaxing and sleep-inducing aromas, like camomile, lavender, marjoram, and frankincense. There are many ways to use essential oils in the bedroom besides vaporization. For an environmentally friendly air freshener, fill a clean glass or thick plastic spray with 1½ cups of warm water, add 10–100 drops of essence (depending on the aroma's strength), and shake. Spray the fragrant water in the air and over carpets and upholstery, but not over polished wood, velvet, or silk.

Use the essential oils to perfume your bed linen, adding 3–6 drops to the fabric conditioner. If you use a tumble dryer, add 2 drops to a cotton handkerchief and place it in the dryer, too. Then store the sheets with some scented cotton balls or a

Make sure that peaceful sleep does not elude you, but comes easily and naturally.

handkerchief to reinforce the aroma. To make sure you inhale the sedative essences that promote restful sleep all through the night, add a drop of any of the light-colored oils to the edge of your pillow. Alternatively, place no more than four scented cotton balls inside each pillowcase, or make an old-fashioned herb sachet to help you drift into a restful slumber. Fill a sealable box with dried hops and camomile and lavender flowers, then add 2 drops of camomile essence and 10 drops of lavender essence. Fold an 8-inch square of gauze or cotton in half, right-side in, and sew along two sides. Turn the sachet right-side out and fill it with the mixture, then fold in the raw edges of fabric and sew them together neatly. Refresh the aroma with drops of essence.

Relaxing potpourri

½ cup frankincense resin

1 cup dried orange peel

1 cup each of dried hops, rose buds or petals, camomile flowers, and lavender flowers

2 tablespoons orrisroot powder

Essential oils: 5 drops mandarin or orange; 5 drops lavender; 1 drop rose or 3 drops frankincense

Mix the ingredients together and leave it in an airtight container for eight weeks. Place the potpourri in a bowl and let the aroma fill the room. Add drops of essence as necessary to refresh the fragrance.

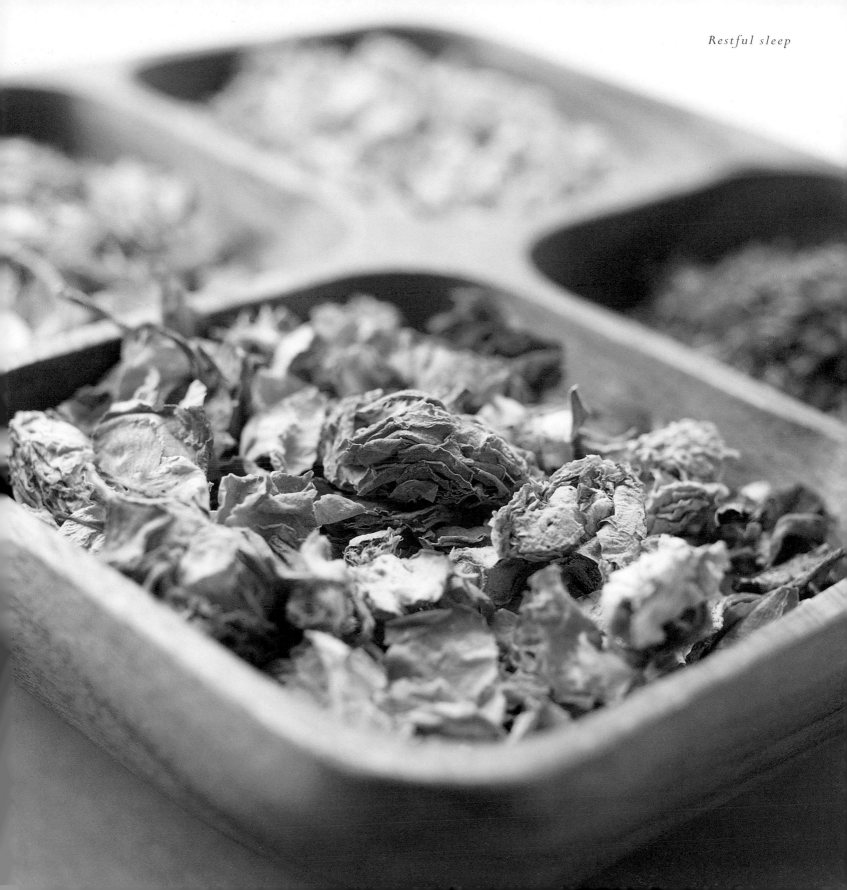

Restful sleep

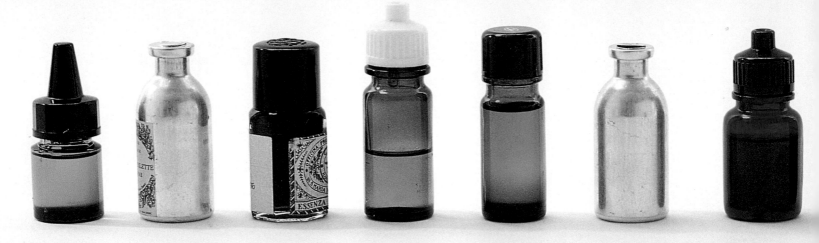

aromatherapy practicalities

Essential oils are safe, gentle, and profoundly effective, but they are extremely concentrated and, as with any therapeutically powerful substance, need to be used with respect. Misuse can result in irritation, sensitization, or actual damage to the system—although this is extremely rare. If you adhere to the following guidelines, you will be able to benefit from and enjoy the essential oils to their full potential.

As with many complementary therapies, aromatherapy works effectively alongside orthodox medicine, and in some instances offers a safe and effective form of treatment for many long-term conditions, especially those linked to stress and tension, such as backache, headaches, sleeping problems, and depression, without the side effects of long-term drug use. Orthodox medicine can provide an important life-saving treatment, but a balanced approach is advisable.

General guidelines

- Before using any essential oils, read the contra-indications on pp. 76–7. Some oils are hazardous, so don't use any not covered in this book without professional advice or further reference.

- Each drop of essential oil is highly concentrated, and the majority should be used only when diluted according to the recommendations. Lavender and tea tree are the only oils that can be used undiluted in small amounts.
- Never use more than 10 drops of essence in a bath. Clean plastic tubs thoroughly after use.
- Do not take oils orally. Serious damage or even death may result if oils are taken internally without professional prescription by an aromatologist or clinical aromatherapist.
- Avoid getting essences in the eye, as this can cause permanent damage. If you do, rinse it with milk and see a doctor immediately. Close eyes during inhalations to avoid irritation.
- Never bring undiluted essential oils into contact with mucus membranes (mouth and respiratory tract and genitalurinary tract), as severe irritation and discomfort may result.
- Certain essences should be strictly avoided during pregnancy, including clary sage, black pepper, cedarwood, geranium, marjoram, and jasmine. It is advisable to avoid using any essential oils in massage during the first three months of pregnancy, and altogether if there

is a history of miscarriage. Exceptions are the very gentle rose, neroli, lavender, and camomile, which can be used safely when diluted: 3–4 drops in baths and 1–2 drops in massage blends. Vaporizing oils is a safe alternative way of using them.
- Estrogenic stimulants, such as clary sage and geranium, should be avoided by women with fibroids, or uterine, ovarian, or breast cancer.
- Lavender, clary sage, and petitgrain are often recommended for treating asthma, but some asthmatics, especially those with hay fever, may find lavender irritates their condition.
- Keep essential oils out of reach of children. Make sure there is adult supervision at all times and give inhalations for short periods only.
- Always consult a medical practitioner in the event of serious or prolonged illness. This is especially important in the care of babies, children, pregnant women, high temperature, convulsions, concussion, and severe burns.

Sensitive skin

- Those with sensitive skin should avoid black pepper, cedarwood, pine, and ginger. Some

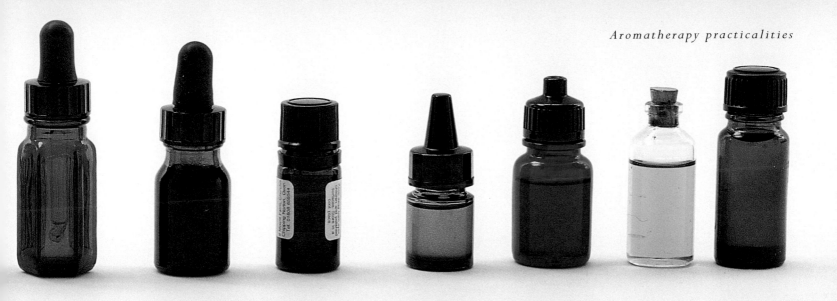

oils act as sensitizers to hypersensitive skin, so avoid benzoin, jasmine, pine, clary sage, and rose, and ylang ylang at high concentration or very regular application. Sandalwood, jasmine, bergamot, ginger, geranium, lime, and vetiver can cause dermatitis on hypersensitive skin.

- If in doubt, do a skin-patch test first. Prepare the dilution of the oil you wish to test, wash and dry the forearm thoroughly, add a sample of the blend to the gauze section of a large bandaid, and apply it to the sensitive skin on the inside of the forearm. Leave it for 24 hours unless irritation or discomfort occurs. If the skin is inflamed or irritated, do not use the essence in question. Although this procedure does not guarantee that an adverse reaction will be prevented, it usually indicates if an oil is not suitable to a particular skin type.
- If you have sensitive skin, dilute essential oils in one teaspoon of milk or vegetable oil before adding them to the bath to ensure adequate dilution and dispersal of the oils.
- Babies and the elderly have hypersensitive skin, so concentrated essences should not be used. Dilute 1 drop in a teaspoon of milk for

baths and 1 drop (of camomile or lavender) in 1 teaspoon of vegetable oil for massage. Or, vaporize the essences or use them in sprays.
- Some oils are phototoxic, making the skin sensitive to ultraviolet light and causing pigmentation. Cedarwood, ginger, and citrus oils like bergamot, mandarin, and orange should be avoided before exposure to the sun or a sun bed.

Massage guidelines
- Do not use more than a 2.5 percent dilution unless professionally advised so to do.
- Do not apply deep pressure during massage, especially in the region of the spine, and do not work on any area that is very painful.
- Avoid pressure on the abdomen and lower back during pregnancy. Only use very gentle techniques, especially in the first three months.
- Do not give vigorous whole-body massage on the first two days of menstruation as it can accelerate bleeding; use gentle or localized massage on arms, hands, feet, legs, and face.
- Do not give massage in cases of the following: severe heart disease; very high or low blood pressure; hemorrhaging, or a history of blood

clotting (stimulating the circulation may cause a blood clot to move); epilepsy (massage with some oils could bring on an attack); high temperature (use cool compresses); serious infection (massage stimulates the circulation, which may cause the infection to spread, and raises the temperature—local application can be used and massage can be beneficial during recuperation, but seek professional advice).
- Avoid the following: site of injury—fractures, open wounds, scar tissue, severe bruising, inflammation, burns or sunburn; infected areas (lavender or tea tree may be effective, but seek professional advice); unidentified lumps (seek medical advice if any are found—they may be fatty tissue, but it is important to check); varicose veins (massage in early stages can help prevent their development).
- Do not massage a subject who has consumed a heavy meal or excessive amounts of alcohol.
- Diabetics can benefit from massage, but only treat those with balanced insulin levels; pay attention to their temperature as they may be insensitive to fluctuations. For those who have been recently diagnosed, seek medical advice.

The 18 essential oils featured are not an exclusive list of essences that promote a relaxed state, but a comprehensive range of the most profoundly calming, sedative, harmonizing, and uplifting oils, which can be used to promote and enhance our ability to recover and recuperate from modern-day stress. Relaxant essences can be divided into five main categories:

Antidepressants Bergamot, clary sage, frankincense, geranium, lavender, mandarin, melissa, neroli, orange, petitgrain, rose, sandalwood, valerian, ylang ylang

Euphorics Benzoin, Clary sage, rose, ylang ylang

Harmonizing Bergamot, geranium, lavender

Hypnotics Camomile, neroli, valerian

Sedatives Benzoin, camomile, clary sage, frankincense, lavender, mandarin, marjoram, melissa, neroli, orange, petitgrain, sandalwood, valerian, vetiver

Benzoin (*Styrax benzoin*)

Benzoin, known as "friars balsam," has been used as incense for thousands of years to drive out evil spirits and to imbue a sense of peace and spirituality.

Physical properties A powerful skin regenerator, especially for dry or inflamed skin; it is protective and helps maintain its moisture and elasticity. The strongly decongestant and expectorant action is helpful for colds, flu, bronchitis, laryngitis, and coughs; it also stimulates urine flow. The warming action soothes muscle and joint pain, arthritis and rheumatism.

Emotional properties Warming, comforting, and soothing, mirroring its physical effects. It helps to relieve feelings of isolation and sadness, dispels anger and releases emotional blocks. It has a reassuring, stabilizing influence, which helps calm nervous anxiety, especially when due to exhaustion.

Contra-indications Can irritate sensitive skin.

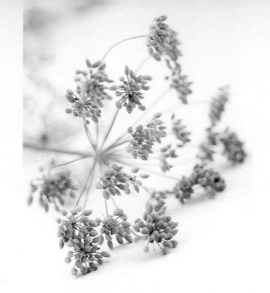

directory of essences

Bergamot (*Citrus bergamia*)

This incredibly versatile and universally loved oil is named after the Italian city, Bergamo, where it was originally sold.

Physical properties Its antiseptic immunity boosting action is particularly recommended for genitalurinary infections, such as recurrent cystitis, and respiratory infections including tonsillitis, colds, coughs, and bad breath. The antiviral and antibacterial properties help acne, spots, eczema, and psoriasis, cold sores, shingles, and chicken pox (in combination with eucalyptus and tea tree). It acts as a digestive stimulant, mild laxative, and analgesic for colitis, trapped wind, and indigestion, and can also be helpful in the treatment of eating disorders and loss of appetite (especially when caused by depression).

Emotional properties Helpful for grief, depression, and anxiety. The balancing action promotes calm, controls anger, and increases self-confidence and self-esteem.

Contra-indications Phototoxic, so can cause pigmentation on exposure to the sun or a sun bed. Can irritate sensitive skin, especially if the oil is old.

Camomile (*Anthemis nobilis*)

Camomile is a gentle oil, so it is particularly appropriate for children. It is very helpful for treating sleeping problems, especially when combined with lavender.

Physical properties A supreme anti-inflammatory that is helpful for dry, sensitive, or irritated skin; inflamed joints and muscular pain; an inflamed digestive system; and burns. It acts as an analgesic (especially in baths and warm compresses) for stomachache, earache, toothache, period pains, and muscle spasm. It is helpful for water retention and irregular periods, and is also a sedative.

Emotional properties A supreme stress reliever, it eases anxiety, nervousness, irritability, and anger. It has a deeply strengthening, calming, soothing, and antidepressant action.

Contra-indications Avoid during the first three months of pregnancy.

Clary sage (*Salvia sclarea*)

Stimulates vivid, often erotic dreams and aids their recollection. Used in massage by some—along with geranium and ylang ylang—to increase breast size.

Physical properties The estrogenic action regulates the menstrual cycle and eases premenstrual tension, period pains, postnatal depression, hot flushes, and labor pains (use in hot compresses). The antispasmodic effect eases muscle pain, cramp and asthmatic spasms. Helps reduce blood pressure, stimulates the circulation, and strengthens the kidneys and genital-urinary organs. Helps prevent dandruff, oily skin and hair, and excessive sweating.

Emotional properties Antidepressant, which helps stress, migraines, and insomnia. Calms and reassures in cases of panic attacks and paranoia, and has a strengthening, uplifting effect for nervousness and depression linked to mental fatigue.

Contra-indications Avoid during pregnancy, with alcohol, and if suffering from endometriosis, fibroids, cysts, or uterine cancer; may irritate sensitive skin. Dilute well to prevent intoxication and headaches; do not drive immediately after use.

Frankincense (*Boswellia thurifera*)

Frankincense has been used for over 5,000 years in meditation, religious ceremonies, health care, beautification, and perfumery. It was used extensively by the Ancient Egyptians, who spent vast sums on importing the resin.

Physical properties It encourages deep breathing and acts as an expectorant, which is helpful for catarrhal conditions—coughs, bronchitis, laryngitis, and asthma. It is immunity boosting and antiseptic, especially for respiratory and genital-urinary tract infections. It is also helpful for skin infections and acts as a skin regenerator, especially for scarred areas, varicose veins, mature, and dry skin—it also has a balancing effect on oily skin. A digestive and uterine tonic, it is soothing and anti-inflammatory for indigestion and diarrhoea (especially when related to nerves, anxiety, and stress).

Emotional properties It is calming, soothing, warming, and stress relieving, and encourages deep breathing and relaxation, so is often used in meditation. Its uplifting, comforting action helps alleviate anxieties, fearfulness, panic attacks, obsessions, nightmares, doubt, and indecision. It helps strengthen positive resolve and a sense of self.
Contra-indications There are none known; it is a very gentle oil.

Geranium
(*Pelargonium graveolens*)

Often used to dilute expensive rose oil.
Physical properties Balances various functions of the body. Regulates the production of sebum by the skin, having an astringent effect on oily skin and promoting renewal and repair on dry and mature skin and some forms of dermatitis, eczema, and shingles. Stimulates the circulation and has a diuretic action, which helps relieve fluid retention, lymphatic sluggishness, cellulitis, urinary-tract infections, and gall stones. Stimulates the adrenal cortex, which secretes regulatory hormones and maintains the balance of sex hormones. Can help premenstrual tension, tender breasts, hot flushes, poor skin, and spots.
Emotional properties Balances emotional extremes linked to the menstrual cycle or stress. Helps mood swings, highs and lows, and irrational angry outbursts. Lifts the mood and refreshes the spirits.
Contra-indications Avoid during the first three months of pregnancy.

Lavender
(*Lavandula angustifolia*)

Highly versatile and gentle essence. A superb treatment for bruises and burns—apply a few drops neat to unbroken skin. Can be vaporized to help cleanse the atmosphere of negative energy.
Physical properties Antimicrobial, antiseptic, and strongly antispasmodic essence,

which acts as a decongestant, general tonic, and immunity booster, and eases muscular tension and period pain. The sedative action lowers high blood pressure, eases palpitations, and calms the digestion. It stimulates cell renewal, soothes and softens the skin, and reduces inflammation.
Emotional properties An antidepressant and nervine, which relieves anxiety and emotional fatigue, balances mood swings, encourages relaxation, and eases tension, headaches, and migraines. Deeply relaxing essence, indicated for those who drive themselves to the point of exhaustion.
Contra-indications Very safe, gentle oil, but may cause irritation to some asthma or hay fever sufferers.

Mandarin (*Citrus nobilis*)

The refreshing scent is a favorite of children and is effective in relieving wind, hiccups, and stomachache. Massage into the stomach in a clockwise direction after bathing, and vaporize. It is also an anti-epileptic essential oil.
Physical properties A digestive tonic, which soothes the intestines and helps ease indigestion, constipation, flatulence, colic, and hiccups. The diuretic action aids the relief of water retention and helps to ease period pains; mandarin essence is often used in detoxification programs, since it stimulates the lymphatic system. It also acts as a gentle immunity booster.
Emotional properties It has a calming, gently sedative effect on the emotionally oversensitive or hyperactive.
Contra-indications Phototoxic, so do not use immediately before exposure to the sun; otherwise, a very gentle oil.

Marjoram (*Origanum majorana*)

Marjoram is an anti-epileptic oil. It should not be used for prolonged periods, as it can diminish your libido; use for specific treatments only. It is particularly recommended for use following a trauma.

Physical properties It has a very strong sedative action and is ideal in a prebed massage or bath in combination with lavender. The antispasmodic action loosens tense, stiff muscles and stimulates circulation in a localized area to release tension and aid detoxification. It eases intestinal cramp and spasm, aiding digestion, and tightness of the chest caused by bronchitis and congestion. It eases period pains and painful muscles and joints, and soothes sore throats and aches and pains related to colds and flu. It has a regulatory action on the menstrual cycle and is also helpful for high blood pressure and heart problems.
Emotional properties A soothing, calming, strongly sedative essence that is useful for emotional extremes caused by stress, anxiety, shock, and grief. It also has a warming, comforting, restful effect.
Contra-indications Avoid during pregnancy, if you suffer from low blood pressure, and in cases of extreme depression due to its strongly sedative effect. Asthmatics should use with care.

Melissa (*Melissa officinalis*)

This is a very expensive oil, which is often adulterated or substituted for a cheaper alternative; if the price doesn't compare to rose or jasmine, it's not the real thing.
Physical properties Melissa essence helps lower high blood pressure and ease rapid heartbeat, palpitations, and hyperventilation, especially when related to stress or shock. It helps relieve nervous tension and stress, and has a soothing antispasmodic action on the gut, so is helpful for nausea and indigestion. It also helps ease period pains and stimulates menstruation. The antibacterial, antiviral, action works on colds and flu, and helps lower temperatures and soothe coughs, colds, headaches, and asthma.
Emotional properties The deeply calming, soothing, and rejuvenating action

helps alleviate emotions relating to stress and tension, nervous exhaustion, and insomnia. It dispels fear, regret, and shock, and promotes acceptance and peace.
Contra-indications Do not use more than 1 percent concentration (1 drop in a full bathtub), as it can have an irritating or sensitizing effect on the skin. Avoid during pregnancy.

Neroli, orange blossom
(*Citrus aurantium*)

Sometimes has a mildly hypnotic, tranquilizing effect. Orange blossom was often included in bridal wreaths to allay first-night nerves and because of the flowers' association with purity.
Physical properties Antiseptic, immunity booster, and decongestant. Good for dry, aging, or sensitive skin, thread veins, and stretch marks. Helps all stress-related symptoms, such as palpitations, tachycardia (rapid heart beat), high blood pressure, colitis, a nervous or upset stomach, and also eases premenstrual tension.
Emotional properties Neroli has a stress-relieving, calming, confidence-boosting effect, and a gently sedative action that helps sleeping problems caused by shock, anxiety, and disappointment. It is a powerful antidepressant, which is especially indicated for agitation and emotional exhaustion leading to the loss of self-confidence and despair. It helps connect the physical and spiritual, and promotes harmony between the mind, body, and spirit.
Contra-indications No ill-effects at all.

Orange (*Citrus aurantium*)

A very cheap, gentle, versatile oil, which makes a wonderful natural air freshener.
Physical properties The antispasmodic action has a warming, soothing effect, which eases aching muscles, chills, and viral discomfort; and releases digestive

spasm, and relaxes the intestines and uterus. It also acts as a digestive tonic, which stimulates the kidneys and gall bladder and eases constipation.

Emotional properties It cheers and revives the spirit and energizes an over-stressed mind, bringing clarity, enhanced concentration, and positiveness. It helps insomnia caused by anxiety or depression.

Contra-indications Phototoxic oil, so do not use before exposure to the sun; can irritate sensitive skin.

Petitgrain (*Citrus aurantium*)

Less potent than neroli, but a fraction of the price. The essence used to be manu-factured from the small unripe oranges of the bitter-orange tree, hence the name "little fruit." The best-quality petitgrain comes from France and Italy.

Physical properties The essence has similar stress-relieving effects to neroli—it eases palpitations, releases muscular tension, calms the digestion, and helps recovery from nervous exhaustion. It relieves congestion caused by respiratory infections and also acts as a deodorant.

Emotional properties Less sedative and spiritually powerful than neroli; petitgrain restores mental clarity and vision.

Contra-indications Occasionally causes irritation to sensitive skin.

Rose (*Rosa damascena*)

Rose is known as the "Queen of Flowers," due to its exquisite perfume and its powerful therapeutic effects on the mental, physical, and spiritual levels.

Physical Properties The incredibly versatile, painkilling, and antiseptic properties boost immunity and help aches, sprains, bronchitis, coughs, sore throats, colds, shingles, and herpes. The antispasmodic action relieves chronic asthma and hay fever and muscular spasm and strain. It stimulates the circulation, helps control palpitations,

lowers cholesterol and blood pressure, helps reduce thread veins, and improves poor skin tone. It relieves hangovers, especially nausea, and inflammation and congestion of the gall bladder, stomach, intestines, and liver. It has a regulatory action on menstruation and eases period pain and menopausal problems. It is also helpful for impotency.

Emotional properties A supremely mood-enhancing essence that helps lift depression and emotional responses to stress and tension. It is therefore helpful for insomnia, headaches, migraines, melancholia, and heartache. It also helps ease impatience and irritation due to stress, fatigue, or sorrow.

Contra-indications May cause a mild allergic reaction if skin is hypersensitive, but this is very rare.

Sandalwood (*Santalum album*)

Sandalwood is the archetypal masculine oil, but can be used by both sexes. The fragrance improves with age and has been used in perfumes in Egypt, China, and India for thousands of years.

Physical properties The strongly antiseptic action is especially effective for treating the respiratory and genital-urinary tracts. Sore throats, bronchitis, dry persistent coughs, bladder infections, such as cystitis and thrush, all respond well. It increases the mucus production of the sexual organs and has a stimulat-ing effect on the production of sex hormones, aiding impotence and frigidity. It acts as a digestive aid, which eases constipation, diarrhoea, and heartburn. It soothes inflamed skin, so is especially effective in aftershaves, and increases the ability of dry, cracked, chapped, sore, and mature skin to retain moisture.

Emotional properties An antidepres-sant with a gentle sedative action, which relieves nervous tension, anxiety, and insomnia. It helps to quieten mental

arguments and obsessions, and breaks an inability to let go of the past. It also engenders a sense of peace, elevating the self beyond mundane distractions and negative influences. Its sweet, earthy nature helps to calm the mind and center the spirit.

Contra-indications The oil may cause an allergic reaction in some hyper-sensitive individuals.

Valerian (*Valeriana officinalis*)

Valerian provided the structure from which the drug Valium was synthesized. True, pure valerian essence is difficult to obtain and is therefore expensive to buy.

Physical properties It helps relieve muscular spasm and tension, including heart pain, palpitations, and high blood pressure, especially when induced by stress, anxiety, or nervousness. It helps relieve digestive spasms and indigestion, and is also recommended for dandruff and an itchy scalp.

Emotional properties Deeply calming and strongly sedative, valerian is helpful for all forms of acute nervousness, restlessness and agitation, panic attacks, hyperventilation, tension headaches, and sleeping problems caused by anxiety.

Contra-indications Avoid during pregnancy. Do not use on sensitive skin, or for babies and children.

Vetiver (*Vetiveria zizanoides*)

The scent improves with age. It can be overpowering independently, but diluted and blended with other oils, it adds an earthy, warming element.

Physical properties Has an antispas-modic effect on muscular aches, sprains, and tension, and eases arthritic pain and general stiffness. Stimulates the renewal and regeneration of skin cells, and softens and moisturizes dry, mature, or prema-turely aging skin, and areas lacking in tone; it also balances oily skin and helps

acne and other inflammatory skin types. It stimulates the immune system, circula-tion, lymphatic system, detoxification, and urine excretion, and absent or scanty menstruation; it also lowers temperatures.

Emotional properties Helps to balance an overstimulated nervous system and lifts depression, mental exhaustion, and insomnia. Brings us back down to earth, enabling us to calm and center ourselves. Protects us from absorbing negativity from others and prevents oversensitivity. It has a nurturing, comforting effect, which can help release insecurity and strengthen the spirit.

Contra-indications May irritate hypersensitive skin, but rarely.

Ylang ylang (*Cananga odorata*)

Can be too heavy and cloying used in isolation, so dilute with citrus and lighter floral oils to gain full glory. Has strong fixative properties that help perfume last. The oil comes in four grades—ylang ylang extra and grades 1, 2, and 3; extra has the supreme therapeutic quality and scent.

Physical properties Ylang ylang calms and strengthens heart functions and acts as a powerful aphrodisiac. Helps lower blood pressure and ease tachycardia, palpitations, and hyperventilation caused by stress and tension. The sedative effect helps insomnia, nervousness, and anxiety, although it can have a stimulating action when used to excess. It regulates hor-mones and adrenal flow, balances sebum output, and soothes dry, inflamed skin. It also acts as a tonic for dry hair and the scalp, and stimulates hair growth.

Emotional properties Balances many extreme emotions—fear, panic, shock, jealously, anger, and frustration. Boosts the ability to relax, helping to relieve emotional blocks and anxieties.

Contra-indications Can irritate sensitive skin; do not use on inflamed areas; exces-sive use can cause nausea or headaches.